PLANT-BASED

for *TIRED PEOPLE*

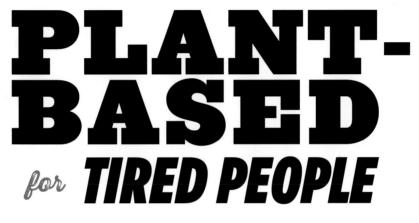

RACHEL MORRIS

CENTENNIAL BOOKS

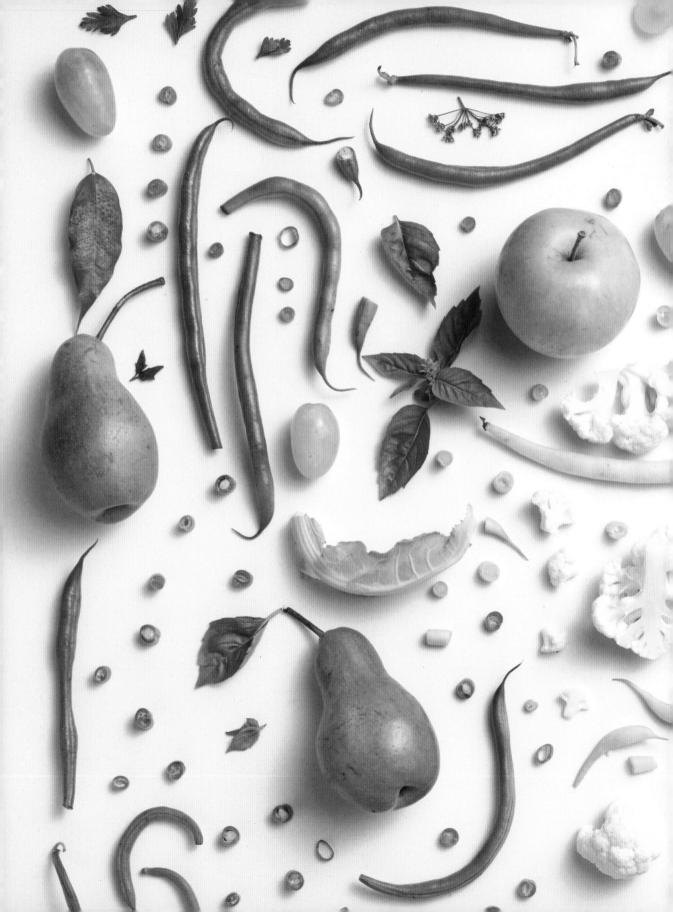

PLANT-BASED
BASED
for *TIRED PEOPLE*

CENTENNIAL BOOKS

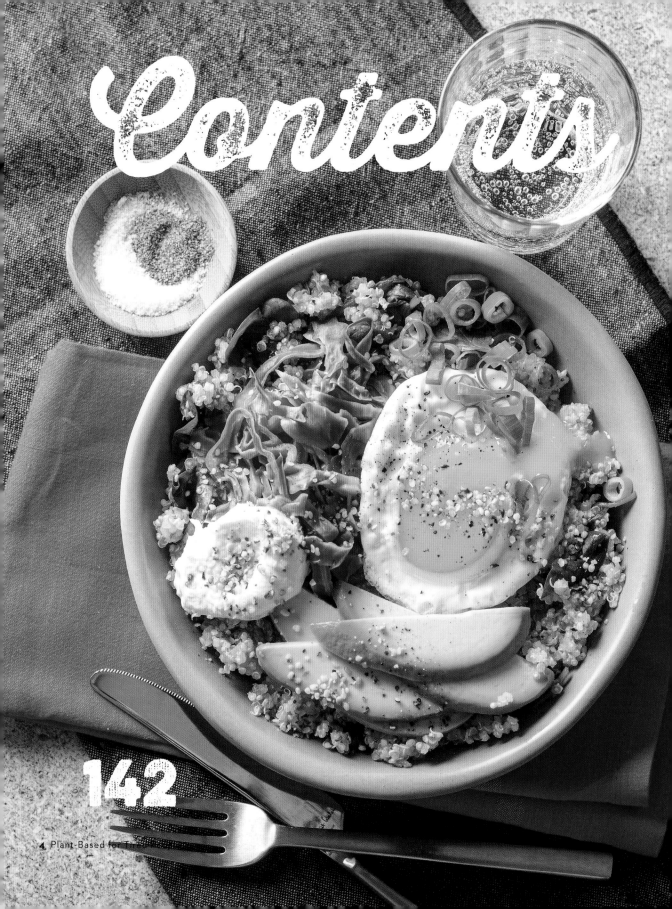

Contents

142

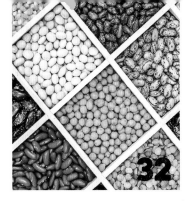
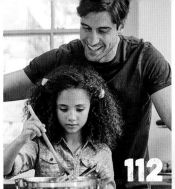
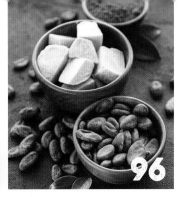

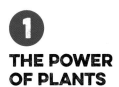 32

 112

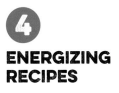 96

1
THE POWER OF PLANTS

2
MAKING THE SWITCH

3
SMART LIVING

4
ENERGIZING RECIPES

The benefits of a plant-based diet go far beyond amazing tastes and flavors!

PUT SOME *Plants* ON YOUR PLATE!

FROM BOOSTING ENERGY TO FIGHTING DISEASE AND MAYBE EVEN SAVING THE PLANET, THERE'S A PLETHORA OF REASONS TO LOOK TO A PLANT-BASED DIET.

Mom was right when she said: Eat your veggies. And if you weren't paying attention back then, now is the time to take her advice to heart. Having a diet rich in produce, along with a variety of other plant-based foods—from nuts and seeds to whole grains—has been shown to be a win for your physical and mental health. And if you're feeling low in energy, plants have some proven power to give you more get-up-and-go.

If you picked up this book, you're likely curious about the plant-based trend. Maybe you're looking for a lasting solution to a troubling health problem, such as high blood pressure or diabetes. It could be that your current dietary choices are leaving you feeling sluggish. Or perhaps, at a time when our environment could use all the help it can get, you may be searching for food sources that take less of a toll on our planet's resources. Could simply changing what's on your plate be the answer? Many doctors and ecologists would enthusiastically nod their heads yes. And for plenty of people who have already gone plant-based, there's no looking back.

As for myself, I became a vegetarian in the fifth grade, when the cow-to-burger connection became too much to digest. It wasn't until a decade-and-a-half later, as a health editor, that I came to fully appreciate my decision. While rooted in an ethical choice, it didn't hurt that my meat-free lifestyle could add years to my life and reduce the risk of heart disease, something that runs in my family. And—the cherry on top—it's a way to make my tiny personal dent in climate change, one oat milk cappuccino at a time.

Plus (and I can't stress this enough) plant-based can—and should!—be delicious. There are endless ways to turn crisp produce, meaty legumes, earthy grains and other plant-based foods into mouthwatering meals that will win you over faster than you can say tempeh. And let's be clear: No one is asking you to give up bacon, ice cream or your other favorite animal-derived products. This is a way of eating we can all adopt. A plant-based diet can be tailored to what feels and tastes right for you: a little less steak here, a little more salad there.

This book will help you figure out how the diet can work for your lifestyle. You'll discover why a plant-based way of eating is more popular than ever, and learn what it can do for your health, including how it can give you a lasting energy boost and leave you feeling less fatigued. Then we'll walk you through the simple steps you can take to switch to a less-meat (or no-meat, your call) diet. And once you're ready to jump in, we've got more than 30 tempting recipes that are sure to become dog-eared, sauce-splattered and memorized by heart.

So let's get started—Mom's going to be delighted.

—Rachel Morris

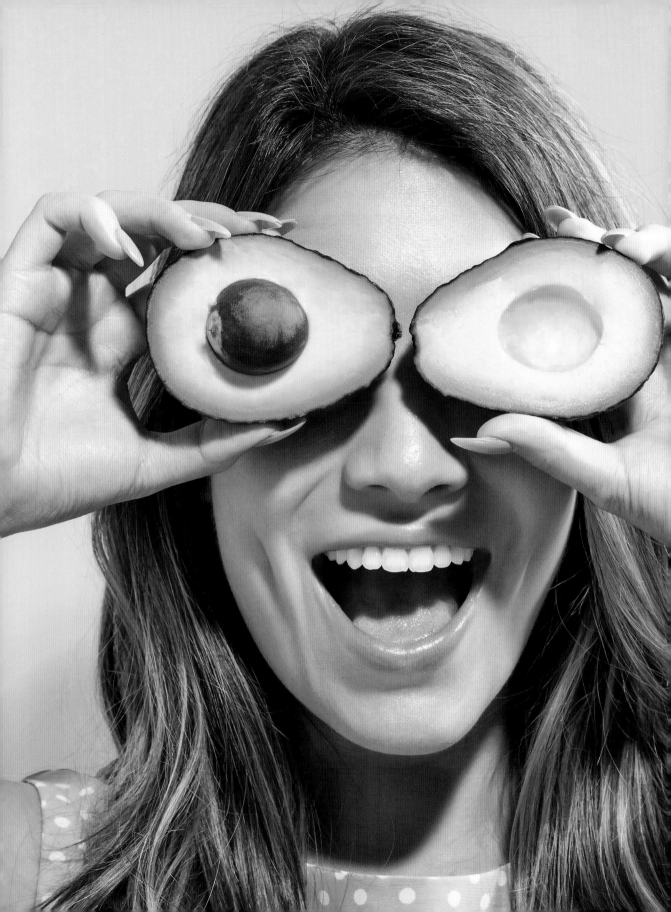

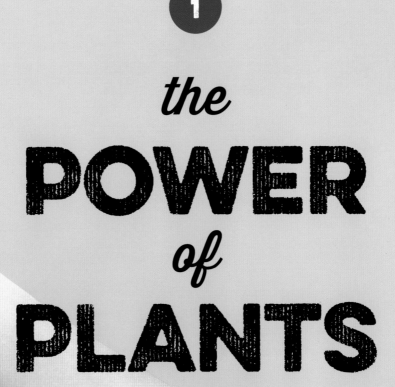

the POWER *of* PLANTS

Learn what this way of eating is all about and discover how enjoying more whole foods can have a positive effect on your health, the environment—and more.

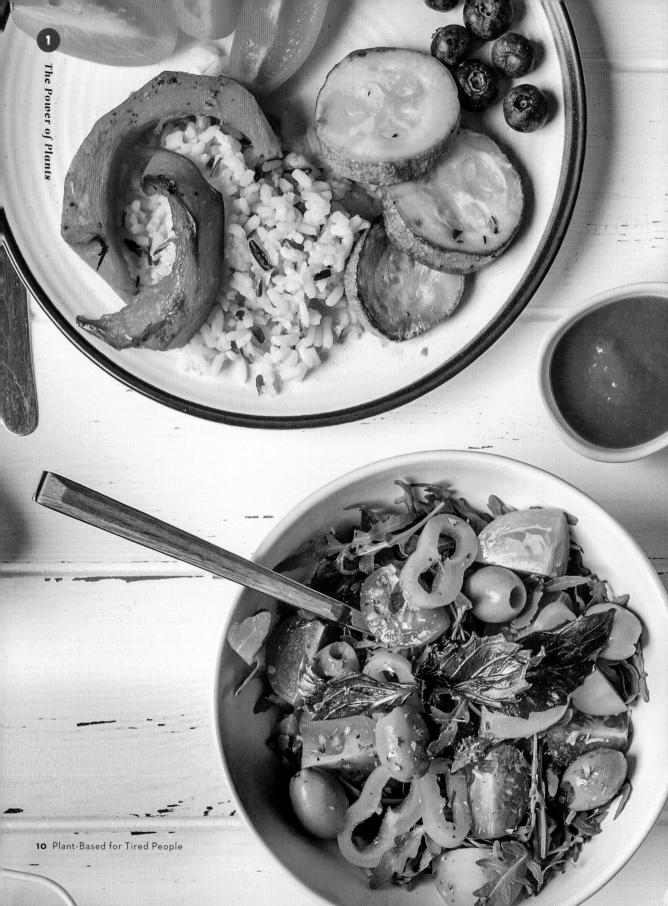

Plant-Based Roots

It's one of the buzziest trends in the wellness world, but the practice of eating from the earth has been around for centuries. Read on to learn how the diet has changed, and what's really involved.

A simple bowl piled sky-high with a rainbow of vegetables, grains, beans and other delicious fare may appear to be a perfect Instagram-worthy meal for our time. But this way of eating predates social media by at least a few centuries.

People have varying reasons for choosing a plant-based diet. Some want to improve their health; others may follow it out of concern for animal welfare or the environment. But one thing is for sure: This is no passing trend.

The Definition

First, let's quash the common misconception that going plant-based means giving up animal products entirely. "The term 'plant-based' is technically undefined," says Julieanna Hever, MS, RD, a registered dietitian, co-author of *The Healthspan Solution*, and nutrition director and co-founder of Efferos. Instead, going plant-based is about eating more plants and less meat—but not necessarily no meat. In fact, research from The NPD Group, a market-research company, found that 90 percent of consumers who buy plant-based products are neither vegan nor vegetarian.

There's no one "right" way to follow the diet, which allows for flexibility and customization—something that may let people stick with the overall eating lifestyle. Someone may, for example, decide to replace one meat-based meal a day with a vegetarian meal, while another person may give up all animal products entirely, including dairy and eggs. They're very different diets, but both can be considered "plant-based." And at a time when so many diets feel restrictive (if not impossible), plant-based is a refreshing—and healthy!—alternative.

Food for Thought

Because there are so many ways to follow the diet, there's no official plant-based food list. That said, there are certain choices that always fit into a plant-based diet, like vegetables, whole grains, beans, legumes, fruit and nuts.

Things can get confusing with foods like pasta and potatoes. Sure, they're both plant-based—but experts say high-calorie, starchy, plant-based foods, as well as processed foods (even plant-based meat alternatives), shouldn't be your regular go-tos.

After all, just because something is plant-based, it doesn't mean it's necessarily nutritious. Just like other processed foods, plant-based meat and dairy alternatives can be chock-full of sodium, fat and sugar, so check labels and, for the most part, aim to fill your plate with whole foods, like veggies and whole grains.

A Brief History

People were, of course, eating plant-based long before the diet started trending on Google. The Greek philosopher Pythagoras adopted a meatless diet, as did Leonardo da Vinci and Benjamin Franklin. But the term "plant-based" as we know it came into play in 1980, when it was coined by T. Colin Campbell, PhD, founder of the T. Colin Campbell Center for Nutrition Studies in Ithaca, New York.

Campbell studied the link between animal-product consumption and increased risk of chronic illness, and he chose his words carefully when describing the diet, avoiding calling it "vegetarian." Said Campbell, "That tends to do with ethics and animal rights, which is great, but if that's the only argument to be made for changing a diet, it doesn't work very well." Instead, his focus was on wellness. "We can actually use this

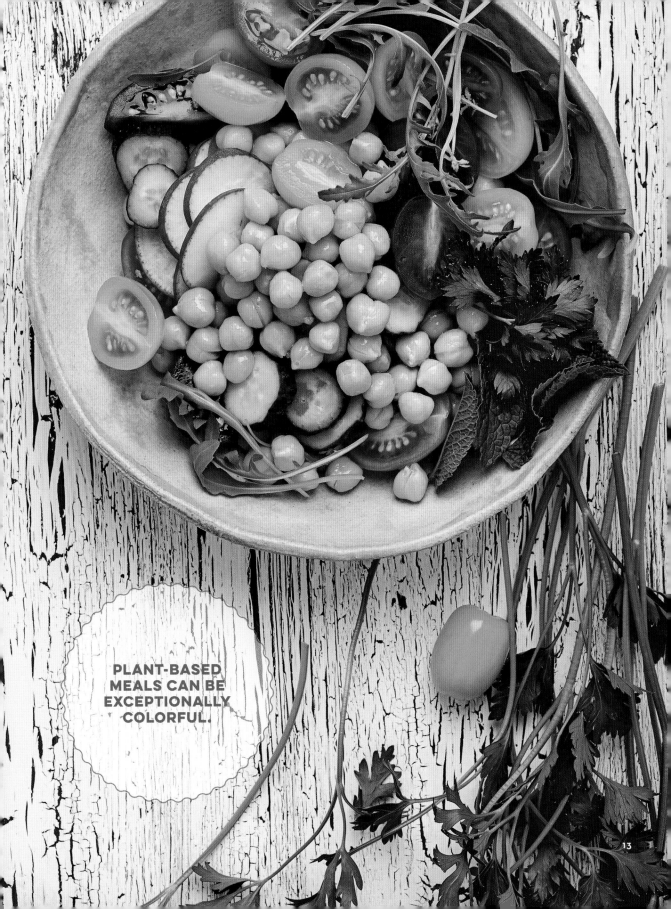

PLANT-BASED
MEALS CAN BE
EXCEPTIONALLY
COLORFUL.

type of diet to prevent disease. And people who already have a disease and switch to a plant-based way of eating can start seeing benefits," he explained. In other words, the diet acts as a preventative treatment and also as medicine.

Campbell hoped the term "plant-based" would bring some clarity to the nutrition world. "We tend to think of diets as how much of this nutrient, how much of that, but that's too confusing," he said. "All we need to do is consume plant-based diets." In 2005, Campbell put his research and thoughts to paper with his book *The China Study*, which went on to become one of the bestselling books on nutrition and has been translated into 50 different languages.

The Current Boom

The past decade saw an explosion in plant-based popularity, thanks in part to documentaries like *Forks Over Knives* and *The Game Changers*, which explore the health benefits of the diet. The flexitarian diet—which encourages eating mainly plant-based foods—tied for second place for best overall diet for 2020 in *U.S. News & World Report*'s annual rankings. All of that buzz is changing what's on people's plates, with one in three Americans saying that they follow a flexitarian diet, according to a recent poll.

In the past few years, the food and beverage industry has adopted the diet, too. If you take a look at supermarket shelves, it's clear that there's never been a better time to go plant-based. Milk and meat alternatives abound, giving both vegans and meat-eaters delicious new ways to add more plants to their plates. Additionally, plant-based cookbooks, blogs and meal-delivery kits provide support and guidance—as do the pages of this book. Keep on reading to learn more about the increasingly popular plant-based diet and use our strategies, guides, recipes and more to find success from the get-go.

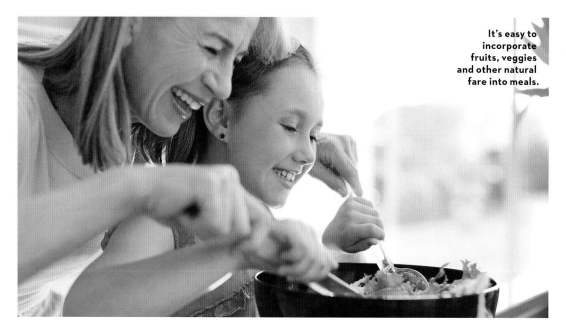

It's easy to incorporate fruits, veggies and other natural fare into meals.

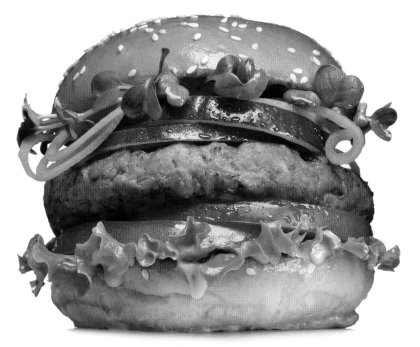

COMMON MYTHS—BUSTED

DON'T LET THESE FOUR MISCONCEPTIONS DETER YOU FROM GOING PLANT-BASED.

THE MYTH
Eating plant-based is expensive.

THE REALITY
A study in the *Journal of Hunger & Environmental Nutrition* found that eating a plant-based diet that uses olive oil as a healthy source of fat costs almost $750 less per year than eating one that is focused around animal protein. And the plant-based diet delivered significantly more servings of fruits, vegetables and whole grains. To further cut down on your grocery costs, consider using frozen veggies and fruit in meals as opposed to fresh—they're just as yummy and nutritious.

THE MYTH
You need to buy organic produce when following a plant-based diet.

THE REALITY
If you prefer to purchase organic products, great— but it's definitely not required. "The benefits of eating more fruits and vegetables far exceeds the risk of ensuring those foods are organically grown," says Julieanna Hever, MS, RD. "Because organic products are not always available and are almost always more expensive, I prefer not to emphasize this as a priority or prerequisite for a healthful diet."

THE MYTH
It's impossible to eat out on a plant-based diet.

THE REALITY
More and more restaurants and fast-food establishments are tweaking their menus to provide plant-based options—a move that's great for business. One report from The Good Food Institute, a nonprofit that promotes plant-based eating, found that when restaurants added more plant-based dishes to their menu, they increased foot traffic, while lowering the cost of ingredients. Many restaurants will highlight vegetarian fare on the menu.

THE MYTH
Plant-based meals aren't filling.

THE REALITY
Even though plant-based meals can be lower in calories than similar meat-based dishes, that doesn't mean you'll be stuck with a grumbling stomach. Plant-based foods like veggies and whole grains tend to be high in filling fiber. If you find that you aren't feeling satisfied after a meal, make sure you're getting enough protein (from sources like beans and tofu) and fat (such as from avocados or olive oil), which will also help fill you up. And don't forget to drink water! Dehydration is often mistaken for hunger.

5 WAYS TO GO PLANT-BASED

THESE STYLES OF EATING LOOK EXTREMELY DIFFERENT—BUT THEY ARE ALL CONSIDERED PART OF THE DIET. WHICH ONE WOULD WORK BEST FOR YOU?

1 FLEXITARIAN
While the diet doesn't eliminate animal products completely, it encourages eating mostly plant-based foods. In other words, there's wiggle room for a burger or grilled chicken if you're in the mood.

2 VEGETARIAN
A vegetarian approach to plant-based means cutting out all meat, poultry and fish—but still leaving space for dairy products and eggs. An egg-and-cheese sandwich totally works—just hold the bacon.

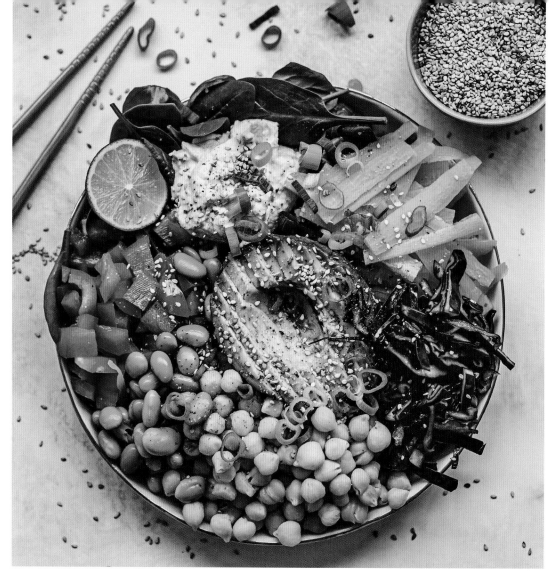

3 **VEGAN**
For vegans, going plant-based means abstaining from all animal products, meaning meat, seafood, eggs, dairy—even honey. Luckily, there's a large number of plant-based meat and dairy alternatives that make it easier than ever to follow this diet.

4 **MEDITERRANEAN**
Traditionally followed by people in places like Greece and Italy, the Mediterranean diet emphasizes plant-based foods like vegetables, fruits, beans, nuts and olive oil, but also includes modest amounts of fish, dairy and lean protein. Red meat is included only sparingly, so when eating out, opt for the salmon and salad, not the steak.

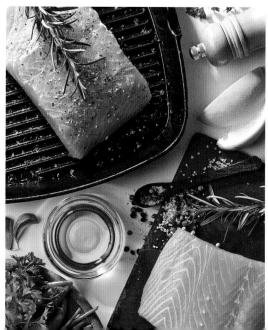

5 RAW FOODS

The food list looks similar to that of a vegan diet, but instead of being cooked, most of the foods are eaten raw. "There are certain nutrients and enzymes that are depleted or destroyed in the cooking process," says Julieanna Hever, MS, RD. "That said, you don't need to exclude cooked foods and remain exclusively raw to benefit. Simply include approximately half or more of your daily calories from raw foods."

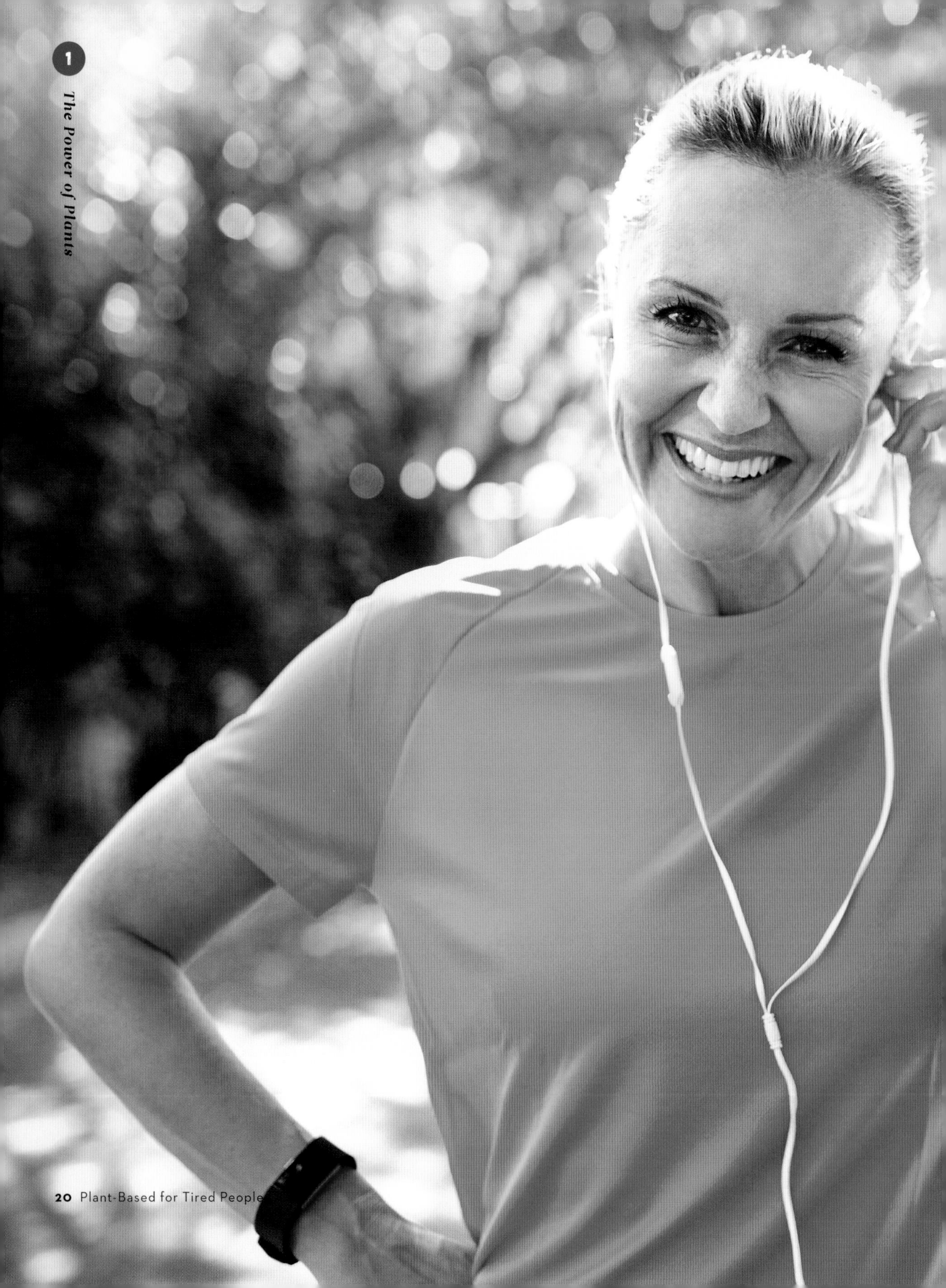

To Good Health!

Going plant-based provides a major win for your well-being. Here are just a few ways that changing your diet boosts your physical health.

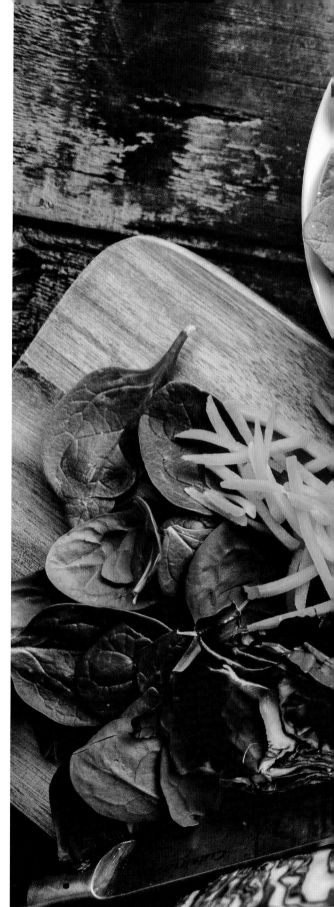

agic pills that improve your health from head to toe? No such thing—but a plant-based diet comes awfully close. After upping your intake of plant-based foods, you may feel more energetic and clearheaded. You might even sleep better, find that your digestion is more predictable, or perhaps feel an overall sense of incredible lightness.

These changes aren't in your head. They are a few of the very real side effects that can come with removing animal products from your menu and replacing them with whole, plant-based foods. You won't need to wait long to get results. "The body reacts quickly," says Ruby Lathon, PhD, a holistic nutritionist and health coach based in Washington, D.C. "We're not just talking tiny steps, but quantum leaps that will benefit you forever."

The Health Advantages

On average, in only one week of eating a whole-food, plant-based diet, people experience a 3-pound drop in weight, along with lowered cholesterol (26 mg/dL) and blood pressure (10/5 mm/Hg), according to results of the Engine 2 Seven-Day Rescue Challenge program (free at plantstrong.com). And that's just the beginning.

Research has found that going plant-based positively impacts the body in numerous ways. The diet can help improve—and even reverse—multiple conditions and physical issues, including allergies and asthma; skin conditions like eczema and psoriasis; gastrointestinal disorders; Type 2 diabetes; heart disease; eye conditions like macular degeneration, cataracts and glaucoma; and cancers of the colon, prostate and breast.

The cherry on top? Research shows that eating a plant-based diet can even boost

Colorful
choices
mean an
abundance of
antioxidants.

longevity. "There's no one dietary pattern other than a whole-food, plant-based diet that has been shown to do all of those things," says James F. Loomis, MD, medical director for the Barnard Medical Center. "It's estimated that 75 to 80 percent of health is determined by the food we put in our mouth."

Why You Feel Better

If you could take a look inside your body after going plant-based, the changes would astound you. When you leave out animal products and processed foods, you reduce oxidative stress, inflammation and toxins that are at the root of dysfunction in our cells and organs. Nourish your body instead with nutrients from whole, plant-based foods, and you are "bathing your body in antioxidants," says Loomis.

Most plant-based diets contain no dietary cholesterol, minimal amounts of saturated fat, and high levels of fiber; these all help open up blood flow in the arteries that can get clogged up from the standard American diet. This healthy blood flow, paired with decreases in inflammation, makes for a healthier body from the inside out.

Meds? Not Here!

The effects of a plant-based diet could even help cut back on medication costs. One large study found that vegetarians are about half as likely to be on medications such as aspirin, sleeping pills, tranquilizers, antacids, painkillers, blood pressure drugs, laxatives and insulin. The best part? Side effects include feeling more alert, enjoying clearer skin and nixing nagging aches and pains. Now that's a doc-approved diet!

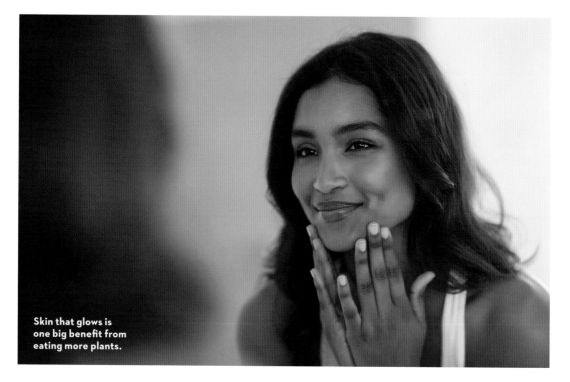

Skin that glows is one big benefit from eating more plants.

WHAT YOU MAY BE MISSING

THOSE WHO FOLLOW A PLANT-BASED DIET—ESPECIALLY VEGANS—MAY NEED SUPPLEMENTS TO COVER THEIR NUTRITION BASES.

If you decide to go all in with plants, you need to be especially vigilant about the quality of your diet. (Junk food happens in the plant-based world, too.) According to Kris Sollid, RD, the senior director of nutrition communications at the International Food Information Council, vegans often run low in the following vitamins and minerals:

VITAMIN B12, also known as cyanocobalamin, is important for metabolism, heart, nerve and muscle health—and it's mostly found in animal products. Vegans should opt for foods fortified with B12, like cereals and other grains.

CALCIUM is essential for dental, nerve, bone and muscle health. It's found predominantly in dairy foods and in lesser amounts in leafy greens like kale and broccoli. A 2019 *Nutrition Reviews* study found that vegans/vegetarians had lower bone density and an increased risk for fractures.

OMEGA-3 FATTY ACIDS are a type of polyunsaturated fat shown to support cardiovascular health. The three most common types of omega-3s are ALA (alpha-linolenic acid), EPA (eicosapentaenoic acid) and DHA (docosahexaenoic acid). "ALA is found in plant sources like flaxseeds, chia seeds and walnuts; EPA and DHA are found mainly in animal foods, with the exception of some marine plant sources," Sollid says. "ALA is converted into EPA and DHA, but only in small quantities," so vegans may need more ALA. Some experts advise vegetarians and vegans to get up to twice the recommended amount of ALA, or 2.2 grams per 1,000 calories. Vegan EPA and DHA sources include microalgae and seaweed food products or supplements.

IRON, a vital component of metabolism and heart health, is found mostly in animal foods. Although fortified whole grains, beans, lentils, spinach and other plant-based foods provide iron, "heme iron, from animal sources, is easiest to absorb," says Michelle Hyman, RD, a registered dietician at Simple Solutions Weight Loss. "You can boost your body's absorption of non-heme (plant-based) iron by consuming vitamin C–rich foods along with it." Try adding bell pepper strips to a bean-based or green salad, or top iron-fortified cereal with sliced strawberries.

* For more information on supplements, see page 126.

YOUR DOC
WILL BE AMAZED
BY YOUR
PROGRESS!

YOUR BODY ON PLANT-BASED

CHECK OUT HOW THE DIET AFFECTS YOU FROM HEAD TO TOE.

HAIR
Anti-aging effects may slow balding, as well as graying.

BRAIN
It can lift depression symptoms and brain fog, and prevent dementia. New research even shows promise that a plant-based diet may reverse Alzheimer's in its early stages.

EYES
May help prevent macular degeneration, glaucoma and cataracts. Many people even report an improvement in their eyesight.

NOSE
You may notice that sinus congestion associated with allergies eases up.

EARS
A plant-based eating plan could help to prevent hearing loss.

THYROID
The diet may balance the thyroid to help prevent or treat hyperthyroidism and hypothyroidism.

CARDIOVASCULAR
Lowers cholesterol and prevents (and even reverses) heart disease by reducing inflammation and scrubbing away plaque in the arteries. Can also lower blood pressure and blood sugar, and reverse Type 2 diabetes.

BREASTS
Studies show that women who eat higher quantities of fruits and vegetables have a lower risk of breast cancer.

LUNGS
In one study, 92 percent reported improvement in asthma symptoms on a vegan diet.

GASTROINTESTINAL
Plant-based foods may control IBS, colitis and Crohn's while increasing the rate of digestion, thereby minimizing the amount of time toxins are in the system.

LIVER AND KIDNEYS
People experience improvements in liver and kidney blood work after only a few months of being on a plant-based diet.

COLON
Red and processed meats can increase the risk of colorectal cancer. A high intake of cruciferous vegetables, such as broccoli, kale and cabbage, is associated with an 18 percent reduced risk of the disease.

PROSTATE
Cutting out dairy may decrease the risk of prostate cancer. A study of men with early-stage prostate cancer found that cancer-cell growth was inhibited after a year of going on a plant-based diet.

PENIS
Healthier sperm and increased blood flow can lead to improved erectile function.

KNEES
The diet can decrease joint pain and swelling that may be due to osteoarthritis and rheumatoid arthritis.

SKIN
Following a plant-based diet may clear up acne, prevent wrinkling and aging of the skin, and ease eczema and psoriasis.

SLEEP
There may be improvements to shut-eye, such as deeper and more restorative sleep.

WEIGHT
Can lead to weight loss, even without adding in exercise or calorie-counting.

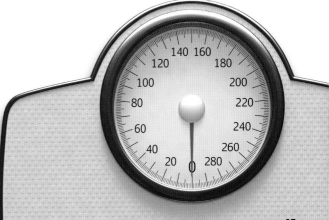

Fired Up

Looking for more energy in your life? Pile on the plants!

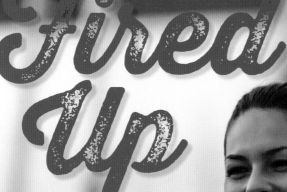

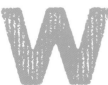

When it comes to getting a little more pep in your step, a plant-based diet is a great place to start. "One of the best things about plant-based foods is that many are rich in complex carbohydrates, which is the body's primary form of energy," notes Ginger Hultin, MS, RDN, a spokesperson for the Academy of Nutrition and Dietetics and the owner of Champagne Nutrition in Seattle.

There's ample evidence that eating less meat and following a plant-based diet can help boost your energy levels and fight fatigue. Take a study published in the *Annals of Nutrition and Metabolism*, which found that 68 workers who took part in a vegan diet (one that eliminates all animal products, including meat, poultry, fish, dairy and eggs) for 22 weeks reported feeling like they had significantly more energy (along with other health attributes like better digestion and sleep) compared to nonvegans. And a larger study of 292 employees published in the *American Journal of Health Promotion* found those on a vegan diet had similar improvements in vitality and emotional well-being after 18 weeks.

A Complex Matter

Carbohydrates are your body's first choice when it comes to fuel. They break down into molecules of glucose, which are then converted into the energy that your muscles and brain need to function, whether you are going for a run or powering through an intense work presentation. There are two main forms of carbohydrates: simple and complex. Those with only one or two sugar molecules linked together are considered simple carbs, or sugars; complex carbs have many more molecular chains and are made up of starches and fiber.

Simple carbs that come from sugar-rich foods like candy or soda break down quickly, which means they can initially spike blood sugar levels, but then lead to a crash, says Hultin. For optimal energy, complex carbs like beans, whole grains, sweet potatoes and quinoa should be your first choice. The fiber in these foods also help to slow digestion, making them a good option when you want your energy levels to last, she adds.

That doesn't mean all carbs that break down quickly are necessarily bad. Take bananas, a classic pre-workout snack that athletes and gym-goers often grab before heading out to exercise. They are an easy-to-digest food that's high in carbs, potassium and vitamin B6, all of which can help increase energy in a hurry. A study published in the journal *PLOS ONE* found bananas even beat out sports drinks in providing energy for athletic activity.

Minding Your Macros

In addition to carbohydrates, the macronutrients fat and protein also figure into your energy equation. "Protein helps to stabilize blood sugar levels, so you don't experience those ups and downs as frequently," notes Hultin. "It helps provide a feeling of fullness and gives you longer-lasting energy." There are plenty of ways to get protein in a plant-based diet, including beans, lentils and soy products, as well as nuts and seeds. Protein is also key to helping rebuild muscles and repair tissue.

Finally, don't forget fat as a fuel source. "Fat is very satiating," says Hultin. "It provides a nice balance to meals and snacks so you feel fuller, longer." Dietary fat has more than twice the amount of energy as carbs or protein (9 calories per gram compared to 4 calories each per gram), so you get more fuel with every bite. If you feel a mid-day lull, try having a snack like peanut butter with apple slices or avocado on sprouted toast for lasting energy.

No-Meat Rules

If you've decided to forgo animal products entirely (i.e., you're following a vegan diet), it's still easy to get all the nutrients you need for energy and good health. But there are a few additional things to keep in mind.

Start by making sure your choices are whole-foods based. Just because a food is meatless doesn't mean it's healthy. After all, Oreos and Fritos are technically vegan, but they won't make anyone's list of nutritious snacks and can often lead to an energy crash. Get the most out of your calories by opting for minimally processed fare like fresh fruits and veggies, whole grains, nuts and seeds.

It's also important to make sure you're taking in *enough* calories, says Hultin. "I often hear from clients that they went vegan but found they were hungry and tired all of the time, largely because they were only eating vegetables and salads and underrating the amount of calories and protein they were getting."

According to the latest Dietary Guidelines for Americans, women should aim for an average of 46 grams of protein per day, and men should aim for 56 grams per day (based on a 2,000-calorie daily diet). But those guidelines may fall short depending on your age, size and activity level, adds Hultin. Another rule of thumb is to aim for .7–1.0 grams of protein per pound of body weight (for 140-pound person, that would be about 98–140 grams per day). Since the body can only break down so much protein at any one time, it's best to spread your intake throughout the day.

Low iron levels can also make you feel listless. Iron-deficiency anemia occurs when the body does not have enough of the mineral, which is used to make the part of the red blood cell that carries oxygen. More prevalent among women (especially those who are pregnant or have heavy periods), the most common symptom of anemia is a constant feeling of fatigue. While iron is found in animal sources like beef and chicken, good plant sources include lentils, spinach, chickpeas, beans, tofu and cashews, as well as chia, hemp and pumpkin seeds. Eating iron-rich foods in combination with those high in vitamin C (think strawberries, broccoli, peppers, kiwi) can also help increase absorption of the mineral.

Other important nutrients may also be lacking in a vegan diet, including vitamin B12, vitamin D, zinc and calcium. Consider taking a daily supplement to balance out these needs (see page 126 for details) or focus on foods like breads and cereals that are fortified with these key nutrients.

Finally, you may want to consult with a registered dietitian, who can help ensure you are meeting all of your nutritional needs—no matter which form of a plant-based diet you choose to follow.

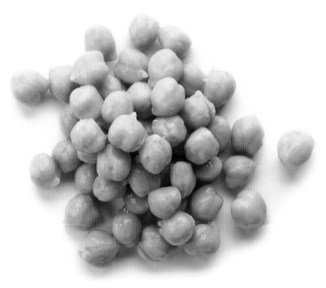

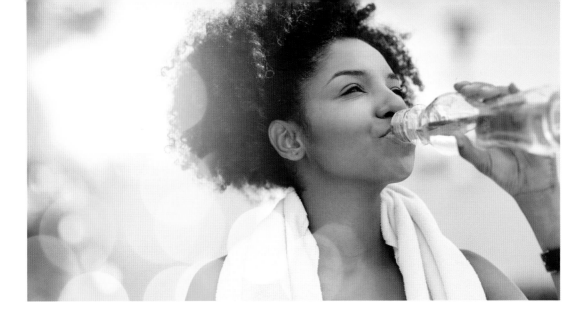

5 MORE ENERGY-BOOSTERS

STILL FEELING SLUGGISH? TRY THESE EASY WAYS TO FIGHT FATIGUE.

1. DRINK UP
Dehydration can often lead to low energy—in fact, it's one of the first symptoms. When you are dehydrated, your blood pressure can drop, decreasing blood flow to the brain and making you feel sleepy and fatigued. Aim to drink water and other fluids regularly throughout the day, and make it easy by keeping a water bottle nearby. Bonus: Plant fare like watermelon, strawberries, cucumber and lettuce have a water content of more than 90 percent, making them delicious options to keep you hydrated.

2. CHEW SOME MINT
Whether it's in the form of gum or a few sprigs of the plant, mint has an energizing effect that can instantly make you feel more alert. Several studies have found chewing gum can enhance alertness and sustained attention. Sniffing a cinnamon stick may have a similar effect.

3. FIND SOME NATURAL CAFFEINE
Sure coffee is a plant-based go-to for a little pick-me-up, but a couple of other beverages can pack an added nutrition punch in addition to their caffeine kick. Matcha, for example, is a bright-green fine powder derived from green tea that contains almost as much caffeine as coffee (70 milligrams in an 8-ounce serving) but with additional antioxidants. Or try yerba mate, a naturally caffeinated herb native to South America that is also rich in many antioxidants, vitamins and minerals; fans say it helps provide the alertness of coffee but without the jittery side effects.

4. TAKE A WALK
Regular physical activity can help everyone feel more energized. One analysis from the University of Georgia of 70 randomized controlled trials found that in 90 percent of the studies, sedentary people who completed a regular exercise program reported improvements in feelings of fatigue compared to those who were more sedentary. And it doesn't take a lot to make a difference in how you feel: Even just a few minutes of movement can help increase energy levels, improve mood and heighten focus.

5. GET A GOOD NIGHT'S SLEEP
No surprise here: If you aren't well-rested, you're bound to be tired the next day. In addition to practicing good sleep hygiene (your room should be cool, dark and quiet) some sleep-inducing plant foods can help you nod off. Tart cherries are high in vitamins A and C and are one of the few food sources of melatonin, which can help improve sleep quality. Or have a bedtime snack of wheat bread with almond butter—the carbs will boost levels of the sleep-inducing amino acid tryptophan and neurochemical serotonin while the nuts provide added protein.

Star Power

10 Foods You Have to Try!

Loaded with nutrients, these "superfoods" will support your health while keeping your taste buds satisfied.

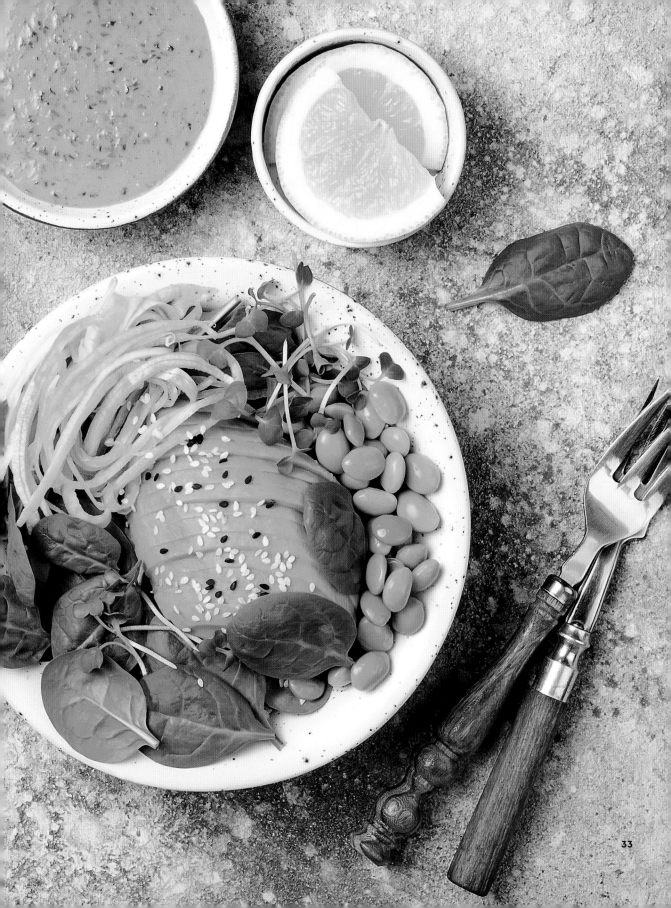

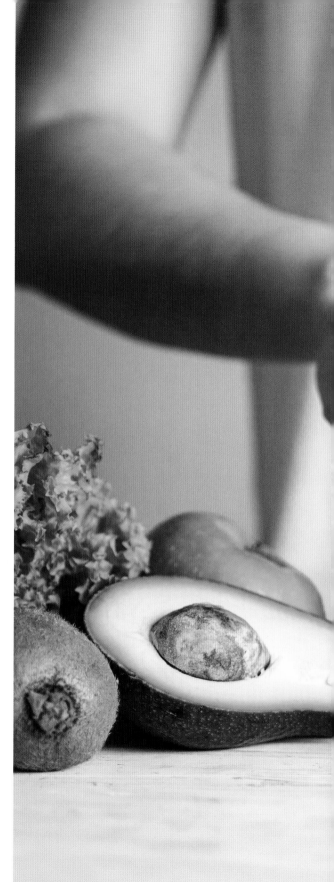

The word "superfood" may bring to mind exotic fruits or funky-sounding (and looking) mushrooms, but you don't have to go on a jungle excursion, scour international markets or spend a ton of money to find foods that are uber-good for you. In fact, you likely already have some staples in your refrigerator and pantry right now that are more than worthy of the moniker.

"A superfood is like a bundle of goodness," explains Keri Gans, MS, RDN, author of *The Small Change Diet* and host of the podcast *The Keri Report*. "It's packed with all these nutrients that have health benefits." Unfortunately, super or not, you can't focus on just one fruit or vegetable to the exclusion of all others. You need variety for good health. "Eating one superfood in the context of an otherwise unhealthy diet won't make a positive effect on your health," she says. "Instead, you have to look at the contents of your entire diet."

That's also why eating food is better for your health than taking supplements. "We don't eat nutrients in isolation," Gans explains. At least in whole foods, they occur along with other vitamins, minerals and nutrients. It's the interaction of all of these together, she adds, that leads to health benefits. (That's one reason so many supplement studies, which look at isolated nutrients, fail to produce good results.)

If you're looking to power up your diet, add the following heavy-lifters to your meal rotation. Each has strong research behind it suggesting a slew of benefits for your heart and blood vessels, brain, gut and more. Even better, they're widely available, relatively inexpensive, and easy to weave into a variety of delicious meals and snacks. Now that's what we call super!

Avocado is a creamy
wonder, packed
with fiber and
healthy fats.

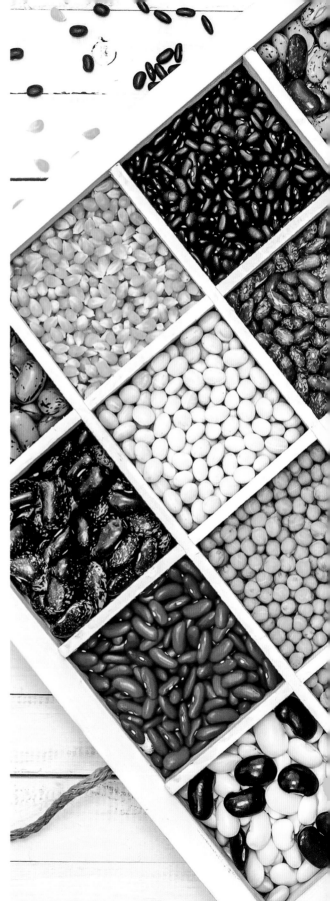

1 Avocado

ITS SUPERPOWER

Creamy, versatile, healthy fats

Consuming one large avocado a day may help you focus better, according to a new study (funded by the Hass Avocado Board). This may be because of its high levels of lutein, a compound shown to support cognitive as well as eye health. The fruit is also good for your heart. According to an analysis of 10 studies published in the *Journal of Clinical Lipidology* in 2016, replacing trans and saturated fats with monounsaturated fats from avocado appears to increase "good" HDL cholesterol and lower "bad" LDL cholesterol.

HOW TO ENJOY IT

Use it in salads, sandwiches, bowls or smoothies. Make creamy chocolate mousse by blending avocado with unsweetened cocoa powder, melted dark chocolate, milk, vanilla and maple syrup.

2 Legumes

THEIR SUPERPOWER

Gut-healthy fiber

Black beans, chickpeas, cannellini beans, lentils, split peas and kidney beans are all good sources of filling fiber and protein. This may be why a meta-analysis published in the *American Journal of Clinical Nutrition* found that including beans or legumes (about a half-cup per day) in your diet may lead to modest weight loss even if you don't restrict calories. And a 2019 review found a connection between eating pulses (beans, peas and lentils) and a reduced risk of cardiovascular disease.

HOW TO ENJOY THEM

Make black bean burgers, use seasoned lentils in plant-based tacos, add them to salads, or roast chickpeas with spices for a crunchy snack.

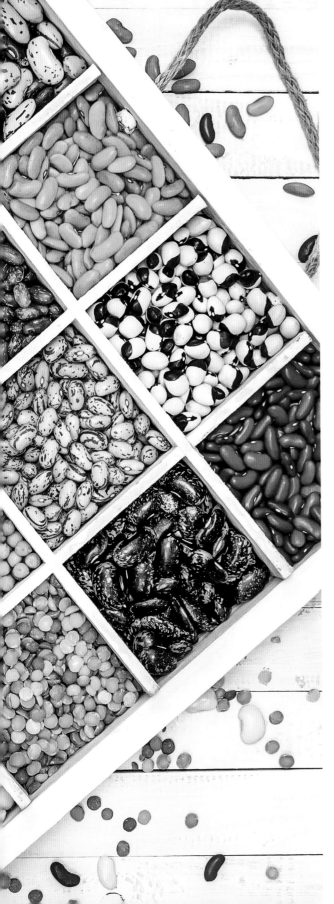

3 Kefir

ITS SUPERPOWER
Probiotics

Kefir is a fermented milk that contains probiotics: "good" bacteria that help keep your gut microbiome healthy. In addition to improving digestion, these probiotics appear to have anti-bacterial, anti-allergic and anti-inflammatory effects. Preliminary research also suggests probiotics may help protect against cancer, but more human studies are necessary.

HOW TO ENJOY IT

Choose kefir with minimal added sugars and drink it plain or as the base in a smoothie. It has a tangy flavor, thanks to the fermentation, so you can also make creamy dressings with it.

4 Nuts

THEIR SUPERPOWER
Compact, convenient nutrient delivery

"Nuts have the triple nutrition win of plant protein, fiber and healthy fats," says Dawn Jackson Blatner, RDN, author of *The Superfood Swap*. Although they are calorically dense, nuts won't weigh you down. Consuming them has been associated with a lower risk of weight gain and obesity over time, as well as reduced risk of coronary heart disease, cognitive decline, Parkinson's and Alzheimer's diseases, and even depression. In one study, depression scores were 26 percent lower in people who consumed just under a quarter-cup of walnuts daily, compared to people who didn't eat nuts.

HOW TO ENJOY THEM

Keep them handy for snacking, chop and mix them into oatmeal. or sprinkle them onto salads for extra crunch. Nut butters also add heft to smoothies.

5 Berries

THEIR SUPERPOWER

Antioxidant brain-booster

"Berries are one of the lowest-sugar, highest-antioxidant fruits," Jackson Blatner says. In particular, two plant-based flavonoids—anthocyanins (which give berries their rich colors) and flavonols—contribute most of the antioxidant power. According to research, eating berries may help prevent and control cardiovascular disease and boost brain health. In one trial published in *PLOS ONE* in 2017, older adults who drank a berry beverage daily for five weeks had reduced total and LDL cholesterol levels, and improved scores on working memory tests. The study authors say berries may help prevent cognitive decline caused by various factors.

HOW TO ENJOY THEM

"Eat whichever berries you like," Gans says, including blueberries, strawberries, raspberries, blackberries and more. They're perfect for raw snacking, but you can make an easy dessert with berries and dark-chocolate chips or almond butter. Toss berries on top of salads for extra zing, and keep frozen berries on hand for smoothies or to thaw and sprinkle onto oatmeal, Jackson Blatner suggests.

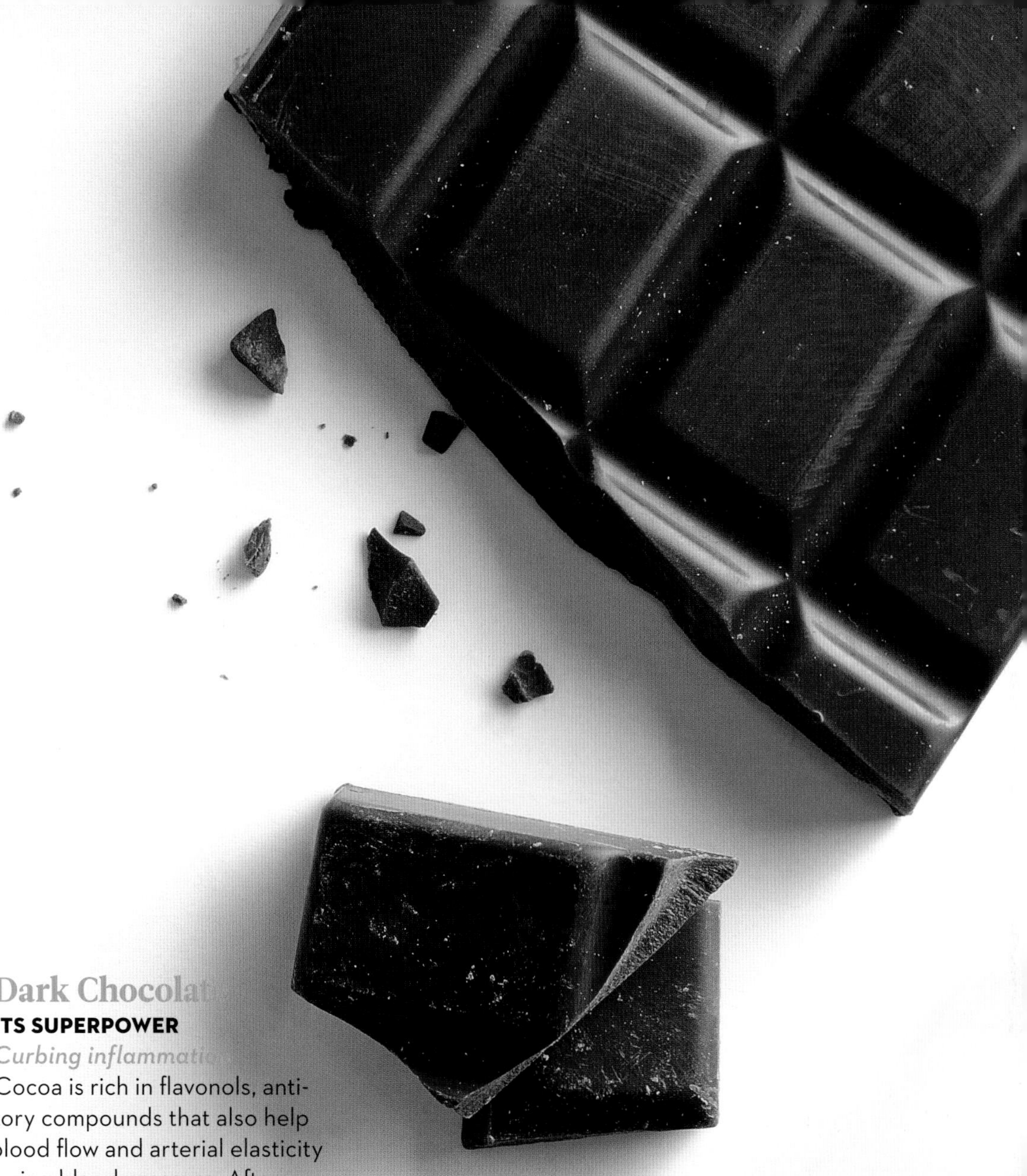

6 Dark Chocolate

ITS SUPERPOWER

Curbing inflammation

Cocoa is rich in flavonols, anti-inflammatory compounds that also help improve blood flow and arterial elasticity while reducing blood pressure. After reviewing 14 studies, researchers in China concluded that 45 grams (about 1 ounce) of chocolate a week appears to be the best dose to reduce the risk of cardiovascular disease. Look for the highest cacao content you can tolerate, which delivers more flavonols.

HOW TO ENJOY IT

"Melt dark-chocolate chips, spread onto parchment paper, top with popcorn, nuts, and freeze-dried berries or cayenne, and freeze," Jackson Blatner suggests.

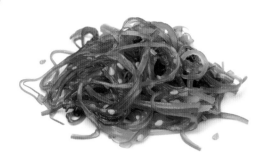

Try making a tea by steeping garlic in hot water (you can cover the taste with a little bit of honey).

7 Seaweed

ITS SUPERPOWER

Regulating the thyroid

All seaweed is rich in iodine, a nutrient needed for managing a healthy thyroid. Seaweed may also help manage Type 2 diabetes, thanks to its combination of fiber, unsaturated fat and polyphenols. In one study, 60 adults consumed an oil containing 1 gram, 2 grams or no fucoxanthin (a carotenoid found in brown seaweed) every day. After eight weeks, the 2-gram group had improved blood sugar levels compared to the placebo group.

HOW TO ENJOY IT

Use it as a wrap, or crumble dried seaweed over salads and bowls.

8 Garlic

ITS SUPERPOWER

Fighting off bugs

Although its pungent smell sets it apart, "garlic is one of the best immune-boosting foods because of its anti-inflammatory, anti-viral and anti-bacterial properties," Jackson Blatner says. It may lower the risk of heart disease and help reduce high blood pressure as well as the risk of some cancers. Plus, garlic appears to be a source of prebiotics, helping to feed certain good bugs in the gut. No wonder it's an integral part of so many recipes!

HOW TO ENJOY IT

Use it cooked to add flavor to just about any meal, but it may be particularly potent when used raw in salad dressings and marinades, or rubbed on toast.

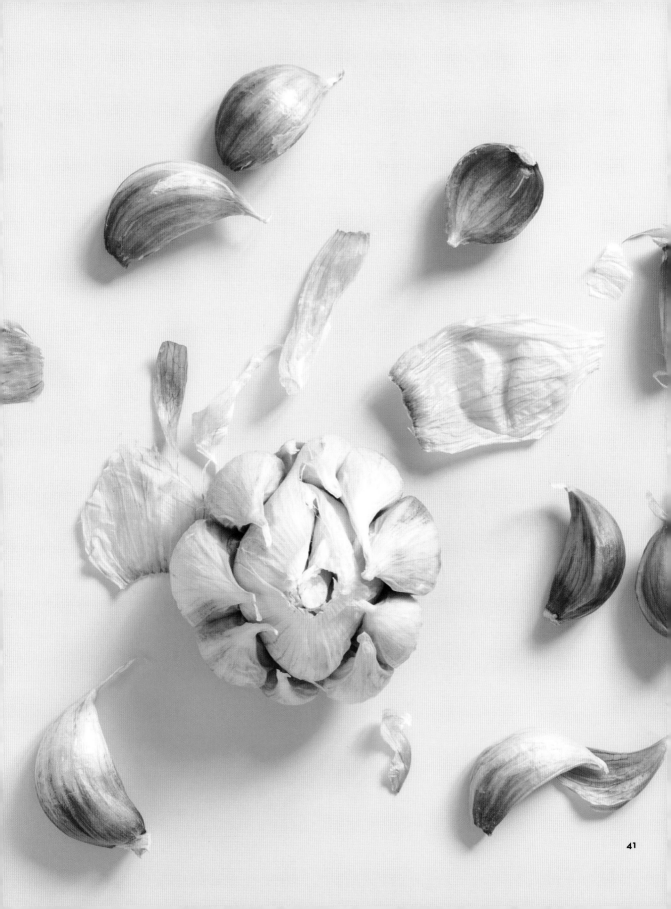

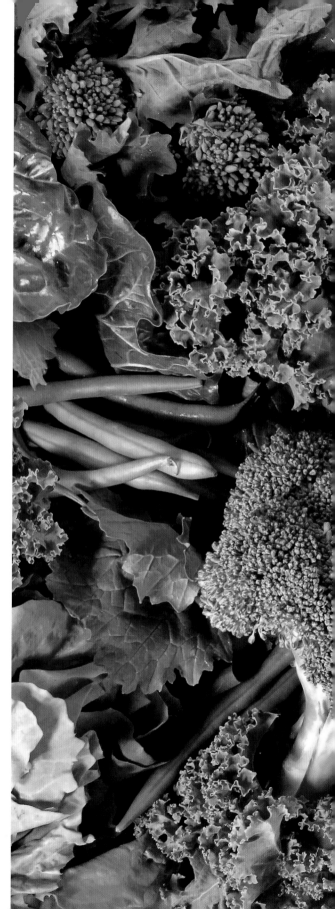

9 Eggs
THEIR SUPERPOWER
Boosting brain power

Don't fear eggs! Research shows that eating an egg a day does not increase the risk of heart disease. Instead, the incredible edible is one of the best sources of choline, an essential nutrient that supports brain health and may help prevent Alzheimer's disease. Additionally, the yolk is an excellent source of lutein—which reduces the risk of eye diseases—as well as important fat-soluble vitamins like D and E, and essential fatty acids.

HOW TO ENJOY THEM
Hard-boiled and eaten as a snack, sliced in salads, or poached and eaten on avocado toast or whole-grain muffins.

10 Dark, Leafy Greens
THEIR SUPERPOWER
Rich (but low-calorie) source of vitamins and minerals

Spinach, kale, Swiss chard, collard greens, lettuces and other leafy greens contain antioxidant vitamins A, C and K, among many other vitamins and minerals. Although vitamin K doesn't get much attention, it's important for blood-clotting and building bone. In a review of eight studies published in *JRSM Cardiovascular Disease*, eating green leafy vegetables led to almost a 16 percent reduced incidence of heart disease. And most leafy greens are relatively low in calories, so enjoy in abundance.

HOW TO ENJOY THEM
Use as a salad base for any leftovers, chop and mix them into omelets and frittatas, add to pasta dishes or fold them into any kind of sandwich (they provide a little crunch). Tip: If you cook greens in water, the vitamins leach out, so use that leftover water to cook your grains, Gans suggests.

SUPER FLAVONOIDS

COLORFUL COMPOUNDS FOR HEALTH.

As different as these superfoods are, many of them have similar compounds: flavonoids. This diverse group of phytochemicals gives foods their various colors and flavors, explains Anupam Bishayee, PhD, professor of pharmacology at Lake Erie College of Osteopathic Medicine.

Because flavonoids are antioxidants, they may help fight off cell damage from free radicals. Additionally, flavonoids appear to suppress pro-inflammatory molecules, decreasing inflammation, and some enhance the immune response.

All of this may explain why a diet rich in flavonoids may help prevent or manage a long list of conditions, including neurodegenerative and neurological diseases; certain cancers; liver disease; pulmonary disease; cardiovascular ailments; viral, bacterial and fungal infections; and metabolic diseases such as diabetes and obesity, Bishayee says.

One study of more than 56,000 people found a link between flavonoid intake and a reduced risk of death from various causes. The sweet spot: 500 mg of flavonoids daily. Aiming for five to nine servings of fruit and vegetables a day should do the job.

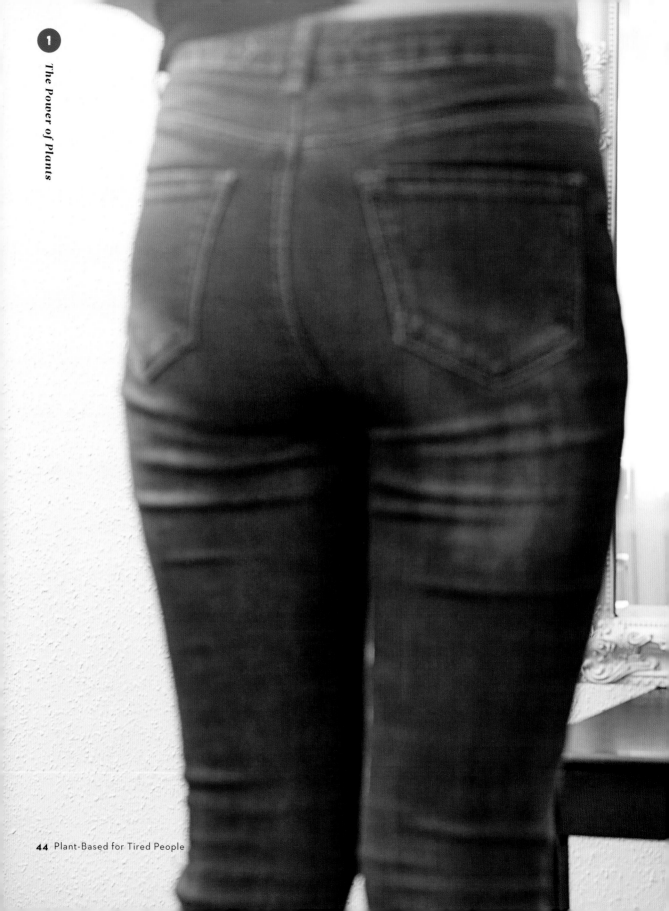

Slim chance

Weight loss is just one of the many possible benefits of going plant-based. If dropping a few pounds is on your to-do list, you'll want to follow these four rules when pursuing this eating style.

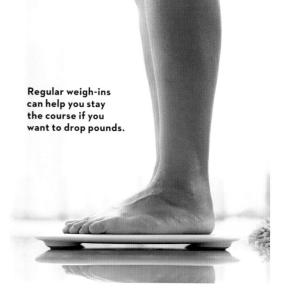

Regular weigh-ins can help you stay the course if you want to drop pounds.

Even if you decide to adopt a plant-based diet for health reasons or to boost energy, you might be keeping your fingers crossed that you'll also lose weight. Here's good news: You likely *will* slim down a bit. Research has found that in addition to the live-longer benefits that plant-based eating can provide, variations of the diet can also help people lose weight and lower the possibility of obesity.

Focusing on plant-based foods may help you curb—or even completely cut out—the less-nutritious eats that hurt weight loss. After all, if you fill most of your plate with vegetables and wholesome plant-based foods, then you won't have as much room in your diet for processed foods, fast food and other unhealthy items that could lead to weight gain.

To help you reach your weight-loss goals while following a plant-based diet, we tapped nutrition experts. Their tips can help you slim down without drastically cutting back on calories—because who wants to feel hungry?

1 Focus on Quality Plant Foods

Reminder! This way of eating doesn't necessarily equal healthy. (Vegan cupcakes and fried vegetable chips, we're looking at you.) "When it comes to eating a plant-based diet for weight loss, I've seen it go both ways," says Elizabeth Huggins, RDN, a registered dietitian at Hilton Head Health in South Carolina. "This is where it depends on the composition of what you're eating."

That doesn't mean chewing kale at every meal—especially if it's not your favorite. It's important to honor how you *like* to eat, rather than trying this diet for a short-term fix, says Amy Gorin, MS, a registered

dietitian and owner of Amy Gorin Nutrition in the New York City area.

"Eating plant-based helps me feel my best, but someone else might say the same about eating meat or poultry every day," says Gorin. "What *is* important is following the basis of a plant-based diet. That means eating fruit or vegetables at every meal and embracing plant-based proteins and healthy fats." These foods can be incorporated into most meals, and will help you feel satiated while nudging you toward your weight-loss goals.

2 Become a Planner

Yes, you can go plant-based even if you have zero cooking skills, but you'll have better control over the calories and fat in your meals if you meal-prep and make healthy recipes at home. Do some research and find realistic, easy recipes to try, suggests Huggins.

It's also important to plan your meals, says Gorin, because it can be more difficult to get enough of certain nutrients from a plant-based diet. Think about what your protein source in each meal is going to be ahead of time—whether that's beans, tofu, edamame or nuts. "I'm also a big fan of nutritional yeast," says Gorin. "You can get a cheesy flavor while adding protein."

Plant foods high in healthy fats, fiber and protein increase satiety.

It's also smart to load up your freezer with frozen fruits and vegetables so that you'll never find yourself without healthy produce to add to meals. "When I'm in a hurry, a frozen bag of cauliflower rice becomes the base of my meal," says Gorin.

3 Fill Up on the Right Foods

Stocking up on healthy foods is paramount for any weight-loss plan, and when it comes to plant-based eating, you'll want to have certain foods on hand to stay satisfied and energized.

Keep a variety of plant proteins—such as no-salt-added beans and legumes, frozen edamame, tofu, natural nut butters, and unsalted seeds and nuts—on hand, suggests Gorin. Beans are an excellent nutrient-dense food to incorporate into a plant-based diet, especially when you're seeking weight loss. One study published in the *American Journal of Clinical Nutrition* found that eating pulses—such as chickpeas, white beans and lentils—daily could lead to a weight loss of close to a pound in about six weeks. That same study also found that consuming pulses was associated with a lower body fat percentage.

4 Keep an Eye on Portions

Yes, this seems face-palm obvious, but here's the thing: Many healthy fats that make up a plant-based diet—like avocado, olive oil, nuts and seeds—are quite high in calories. Portion awareness is critical for weight loss, says Huggins. Look at food-nutrition labels to determine portion sizes before chowing down, and use a food scale or measuring cups to check what a portion size *actually* looks like. You may be pouring out more calories than you think!

One cup of edamame has 17 grams of protein and 8 grams of fiber.

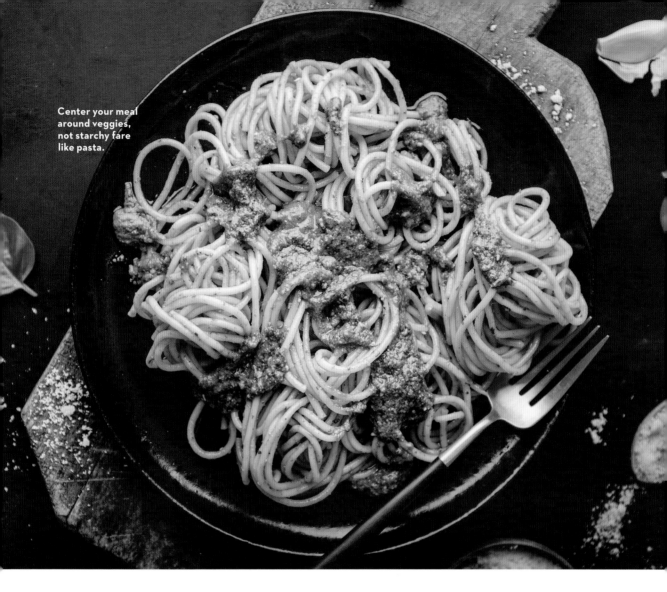

Center your meal around veggies, not starchy fare like pasta.

PITFALLS TO AVOID

THESE HABITS CAN GET IN THE WAY OF WEIGHT LOSS.

OVERDOING IT ON CARBS
"A plant-based diet isn't necessarily low-calorie or balanced," says Amy Gorin, MS. You can eat a huge plate of pasta every night with French fries—but that meal isn't balanced, and it won't help you with weight loss. Start with vegetables and build from there.

NOT EATING ENOUGH
"I find that some clients on a plant-based plan eat a meal that's too light earlier in the day, then they're starving when they get home from work," says Elizabeth Huggins, RDN. That can set you up for overeating the wrong foods later. If you find that your go-to meals aren't keeping you full, bulk them up!

DRINKING YOUR CALORIES
From kombucha to coconut water, sipping on too many beverages friendly to plant-based eating can add extra calories to your diet. If you suspect that drinks could be holding you back, aim to drink water the majority of the time (you can add fruit slices to jazz up plain H2O).

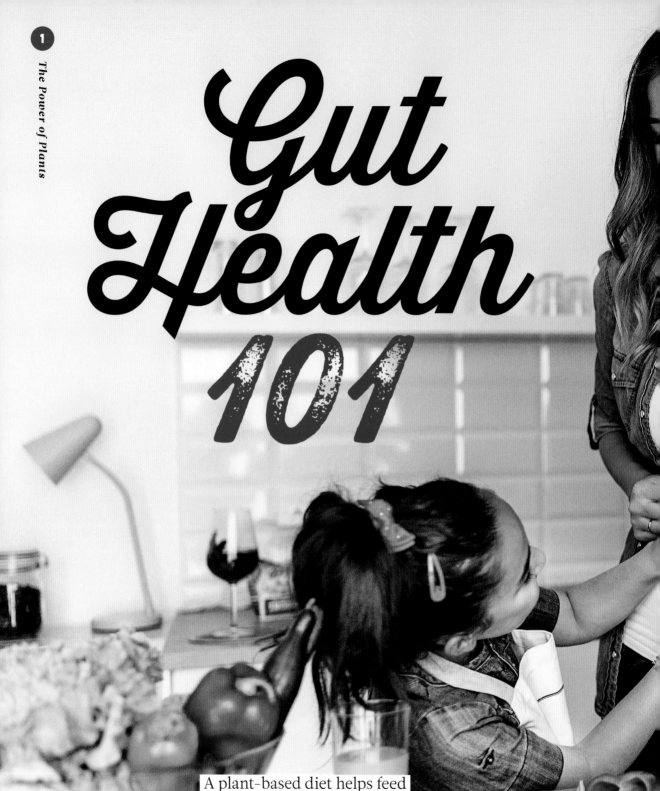

Gut Health 101

A plant-based diet helps feed
the good-for-you bugs in your belly.

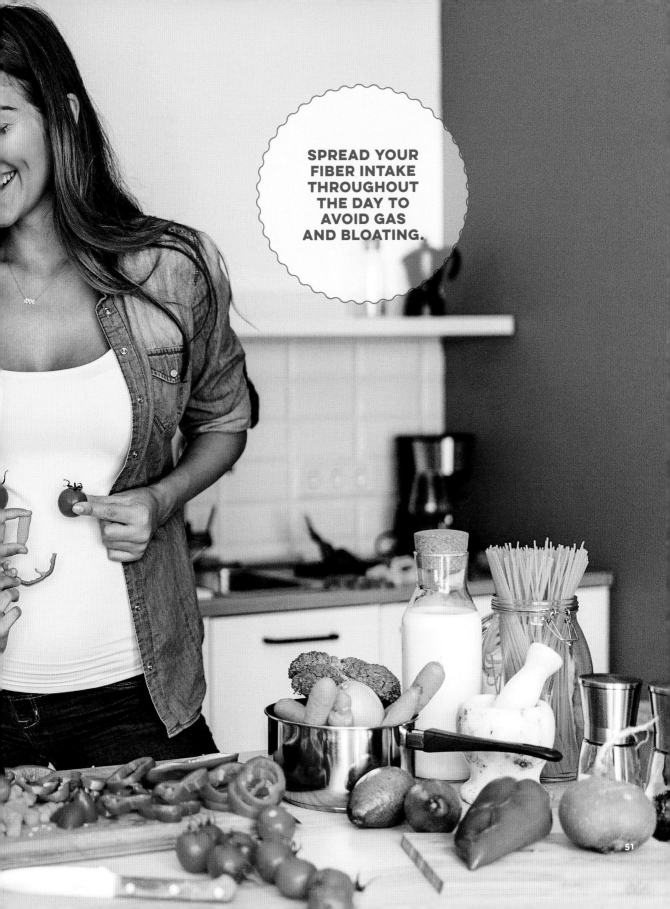

SPREAD YOUR
FIBER INTAKE
THROUGHOUT
THE DAY TO
AVOID GAS
AND BLOATING.

igestion may seem like a pretty straightforward process: Food goes in, makes its way through what is essentially a long, hollow tube, and within a day or so goes out. The GI tract is like a chop shop, stripping down whatever you put in—tofu, avocado or a doughnut—into "parts," the various nutrients that your body needs to survive. It's incredibly nuanced, a finely tuned and timed interplay involving a variety of organs, hormones, enzymes and neurotransmitters. And a plant-based diet can have a big impact on how well it works.

Digestion starts in the mouth and continues in the stomach before food gets sent, bit by bit, to the small intestine, where the absorption of carbs, fat and protein occurs along a 20-foot stretch. Some food, like fiber, doesn't get broken down in the small intestine; it goes right on through to the 5-foot-long stretch of the large intestine. Here, trillions of bacteria munch away on certain types of fiber. The result of that smorgasbord: compounds (sometimes called postbiotics) that affect all sorts of processes in the body. After 12 to 24 hours, whatever remains is shuttled out in the feces (which is mostly water as well as bacteria, protein, carbohydrates and fat).

Cross-Talk

But the biota in your colon aren't just affected by food. Hormonal shifts, stress, allergies, circadian rhythms, drugs and more can all impact the gut and disrupt the population of bugs residing there. Chronically stressed? The signals between your brain and bowel can lead to constipation, abdominal pain and more. Sleep-deprived? It throws off the microbiome and makes you crave food that will feed unwelcome bugs. Diets high in sugar and refined foods—and lacking fiber—create "dysbiosis," an imbalance in the good-to-bad bug ratio. That can lead to gas, bloating and stomach upset as well as depression, anxiety, exacerbated stress and more. If things get too bad, the bugs may start munching on the lining of your intestines, leading to what's called intestinal permeability or "leaky gut" syndrome. That can trigger more systemic issues, like inflammation and autoimmune disorders.

"There are so many things that can be impacted by the gut," says Kim Kulp, RDN, a dietitian in private practice in the San Francisco Bay area. "It's those mystery problems that nobody can figure out that can be tied to gut health. I look at what my clients are eating and try to see the connection. Mental health has been shown in the research to be impacted by the gut, as well as autoimmune diseases."

It's not all bad news. Healthy habits like mindfulness, good sleep and exercise—and of course, diet—boost the beneficial bug population. These habits are the foundation of good health, perhaps because they have such a positive effect on the digestive system.

Feed Your Critters

In order to get good postbiotics, you need to put in good prebiotics. Prebiotics are food for the bacteria that have been shown to have a health benefit, says Kulp. They're primarily dietary fiber, but certain foods are thought to be especially appealing to the bugs, including Jerusalem artichokes, onions, garlic, bananas and dark leafy greens. "Fruits and vegetables, but also whole grains, beans and nuts and seeds—and a variety of all of these—is really what the research is showing works best for producing the greatest variety of gut bugs," Kulp adds. "And that's connected to better health."

Fiber All-Stars

GREEN PEAS
(9 g per cup)

LENTILS
(8 g per cup)

RASPBERRIES
(8 g per cup)

BLACK BEANS
(7.5 g per cup)

WHOLE-WHEAT PASTA
(6 g per cup)

CHIA SEEDS
(5 g per cup)

PEAR
(5 g per medium pear)

BROCCOLI
(5 g per cup)

BRAN FLAKES
(5 g per cup)

QUINOA
(5 g per cup)

APPLE
(4.5 g per medium apple, with skin on)

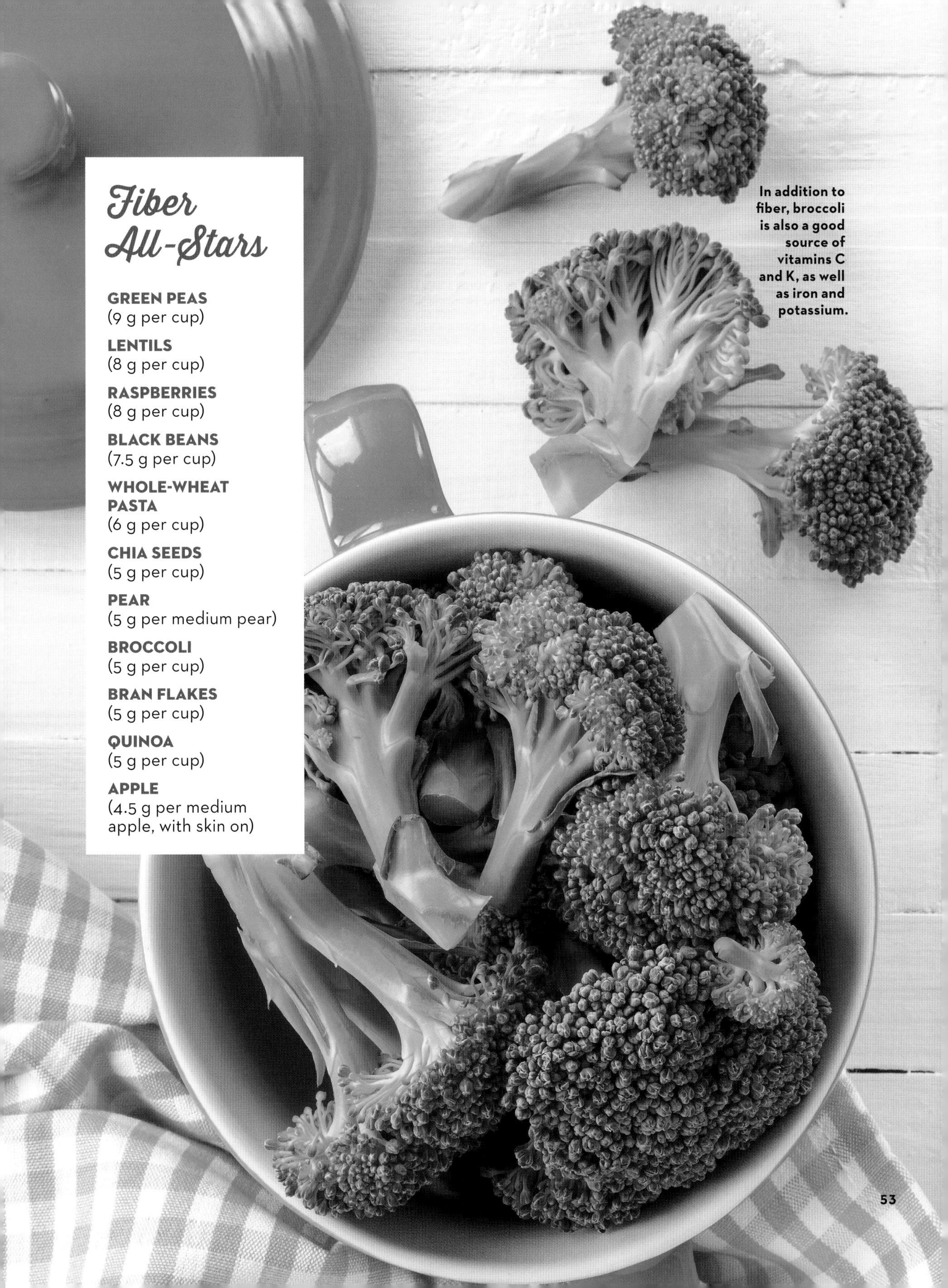

In addition to fiber, broccoli is also a good source of vitamins C and K, as well as iron and potassium.

You've probably heard about probiotic foods, which contain live bacteria that help repopulate the health-promoting communities in your gut. Probiotics are undoubtedly important, but research is still trying to figure out how they affect the critters inside you. While fermented foods do contain bacteria, "all fermented foods do not automatically contain probiotics," says Kulp. "In order for a food to be considered probiotic, it has to contain live bacteria that clinical research has shown confer a health benefit." Right now there's only research showing yogurt (with live cultures) and kefir (a fermented milk drink) are beneficial, but other types of fermented foods—miso, kimchi, kombucha, sauerkraut

and tempeh—may have benefits and are healthy to eat as well.

You can also buy probiotic supplements, but there's just not enough research showing which strains of bacteria work for which people, since everyone has a different microbiome makeup. Some probiotic supplements may not even make it to the large intestine.

The gut is still a bit like the wild, wild West. There's so much to look at and it's difficult to do on live people (most gut research is conducted in mice or rats). Lifestyle changes and diet are the easiest ways to try to suss out what may be causing issues, and they are likely to be the first things that your doctor will recommend.

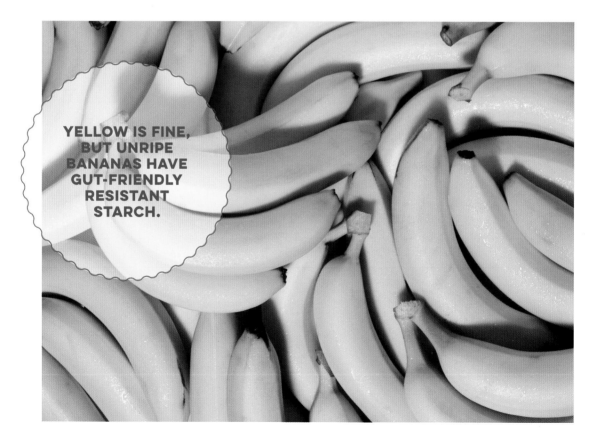

YELLOW IS FINE, BUT UNRIPE BANANAS HAVE GUT-FRIENDLY RESISTANT STARCH.

THE GUT'S CONNECTED TO...

**RESEARCHERS HAVE FOUND STRONG LINKS (CALLED AXES) BETWEEN
THE FOLLOWING PARTS OF THE BODY AND THE GI MICROBIOME.**

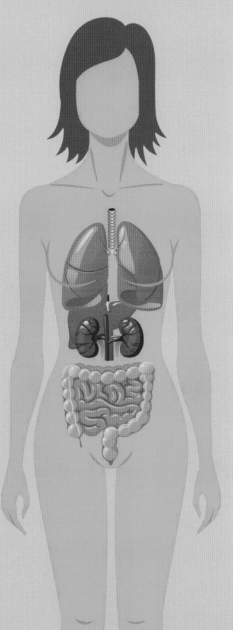

...THE LUNGS
Research has shown how microbes in the lungs communicate with those in the gut, and how the latter are key for fighting off bacterial invaders in the lungs, like certain types of pneumonia. Reduced microbiome diversity has been associated with asthma and COPD.

...THE LIVER
Various liver diseases have been linked with dysbiosis, an imbalance in good-to-bad microbes. Rates of nonalcoholic fatty liver disease (NAFLD)—which occurs when fat infiltrates this crucial organ—are rising rapidly among kids and adults.

...THE SKIN
A 2018 review study found skin issues like acne, dermatitis and eczema may be a result of an inflammatory response caused by microbes in the GI tract.

...THE BRAIN
Fascinating research has shown there's an active two-way connection between the brain and belly. The microbiome can trigger changes in the brain, via the vagus nerve, that may lead to depression and anxiety, and these conditions can impact the bugs in your belly as well. Some studies have shown people with Alzheimer's have less microbial diversity than those who do not have dementia.

...ESTROGEN AND THE REPRODUCTIVE TRACT
A 2017 review in *Maturitas* evaluated the many ways microbial dysbiosis negatively impacts estrogen circulation and how this may contribute to cancer; metabolic syndrome; menopausal symptoms like hot flashes; heart disease; PCOS (polycystic ovary syndrome); endometriosis and more.

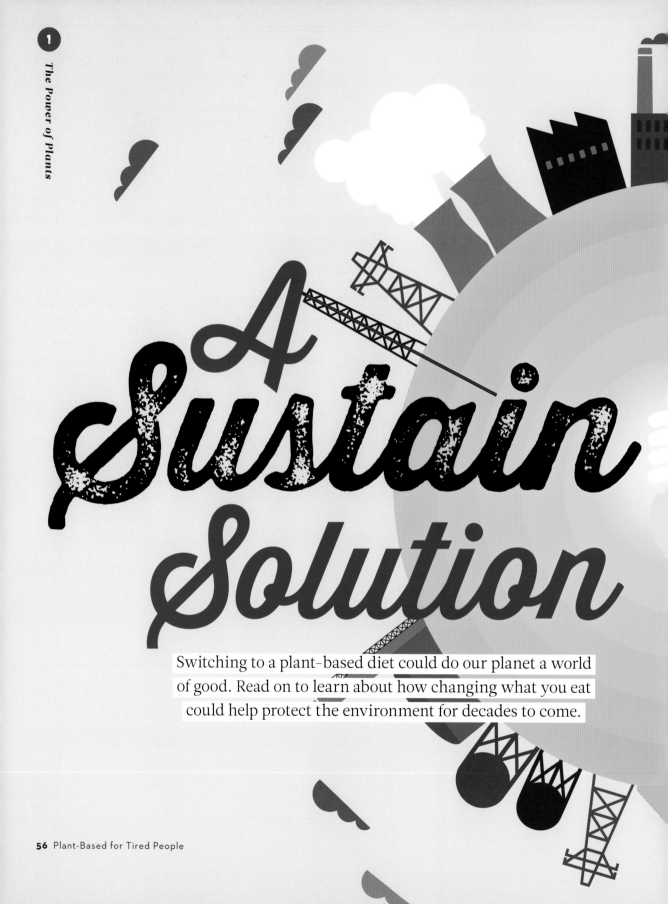

A Sustain Solution

Switching to a plant-based diet could do our planet a world of good. Read on to learn about how changing what you eat could help protect the environment for decades to come.

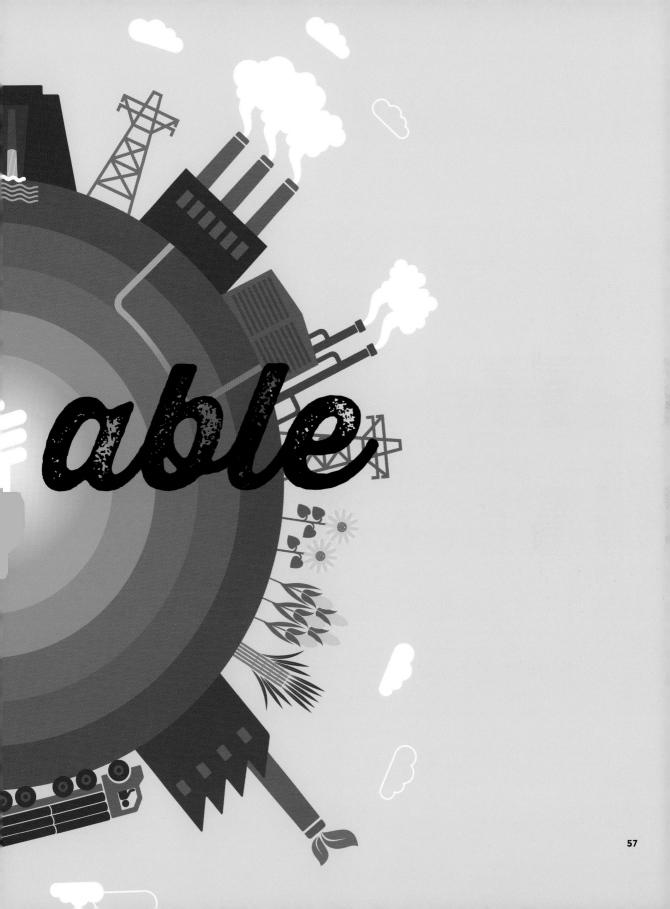

The threat is real. Research shows that if the current predominant global diet—one that's high in meats, sugars, refined fats and oils—continues unchecked, it will contribute to about 80 percent of global agricultural greenhouse-gas emissions by 2050. In fact, livestock accounts for 77 percent of global farming land but only produces 18 percent of the world's calories and 37 percent of its total protein, according to a 2020 report. But there's hope: Changing the way we produce and consume food can slow down this scary trend. From using less water to preserving land and more, plant-based eating is a good way to love Mother Earth.

What's Happening?

The greenhouse effect is natural—and necessary! But it's also contributing to climate change. Here's the play-by-play:

1. When solar radiation reaches the Earth, it's reflected back into space.

2. A portion of this heat escapes, but greenhouse gases in the atmosphere (like carbon dioxide, methane and nitrous oxide) trap some of it. This keeps our planet warm, allowing life to exist.

3. Human activity—like burning fossil fuels and clearing land for farming—increases the amount of greenhouse gases on Earth.

4. The extra gases lead to more heat being trapped, making the planet dangerously warm (aka climate change).

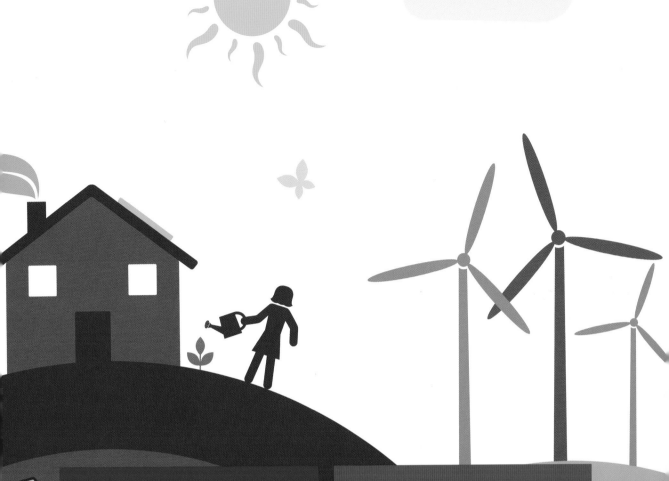

Cause for Concern

● As incomes increased between 1961 and 2009, people began eating more meat.

● One serving of beef causes more greenhouse gas emissions than 20 servings of vegetables.

● Animals require a lot of food. It takes 13 pounds of grain to produce 1 pound of beef.

● Water worry: 70 percent of freshwater use is guzzled up by agriculture.

● It takes about 1,800 gallons of water to produce just 1 pound of beef.

● Meanwhile...780 million people worldwide don't have access to safe drinking water.

Why Plant-Based Diets Can Help

● The farming involved for plant-based diets requires fewer natural resources.

● If the world adopted plant-based diets, greenhouse gas emissions would be cut by an amount equal to the current combined emissions of all cars, trucks, planes, trains and ships.

● Fruit- and veggie-heavy diets require less use of land, which could prevent environmental destruction of an area that's as large as half of the United States.

● If someone who eats 3.5 ounces of meat daily cuts their intake in half, their carbon footprint would shrink 35 percent.

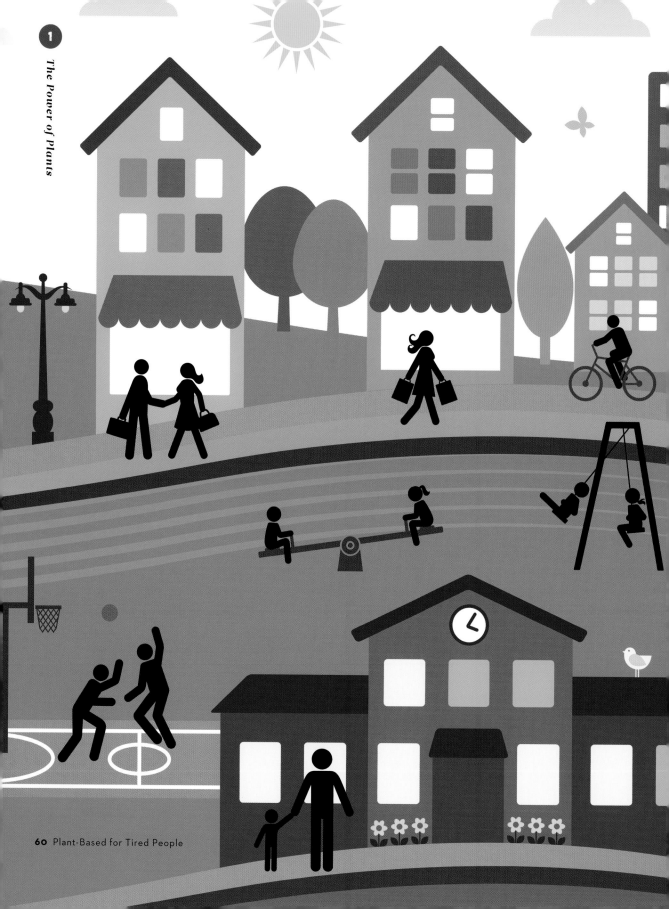

10 MORE WAYS TO HELP THE EARTH

IT DOESN'T TAKE MUCH TO MAKE A DIFFERENCE.
HERE, SOME SIMPLE WAYS YOU CAN HAVE A POSITIVE IMPACT ON THE ENVIRONMENT.

1. SWAP OUT YOUR LIGHT BULBS
Replace traditional incandescent light bulbs with light emitting diodes (LEDs). Besides being more cost-effective, the LED versions use 75 to 80 percent less energy.

2. REPLACE DISPOSABLE PLASTICS WITH REUSABLE ONES
Up to 80 percent of the pollution in the ocean comes from plastic straws, bags and other one-time-use plastic products, reports environmental nonprofit group Ocean Conservancy. They also often contain harmful chemicals like BPA, which can affect wildlife—and humans.

3. TAKE UP COMPOSTING
Food scraps and yard waste make up more than 28 percent of what we send to landfills, according to the Environmental Protection Agency. Transform that waste into soil and kick-start a flourishing garden by combining materials like dead leaves, branches and twigs with grass clippings, vegetable waste, fruit scraps and coffee grounds. (For how to get started, go to epa.gov.)

4. INSTALL LOW-FLOW BATHROOM APPLIANCES
Both low-flow shower heads and low-flow toilets can reduce your home's water use immensely— about 25 to 60 percent in water savings for each shower head and water-efficient toilet, according to the U.S. Department of Energy.

5. THROW A CARPET ON THE FLOOR
Heating accounts for almost half of the average household utility bill, according to the U.S. Department of Energy, and a home can lose up to 20 percent of its heat through uninsulated flooring. Placing carpets and throw rugs on the floor—especially when combined with energy-efficient pads—can curb heating costs, and keep you warmer in the winter.

6. UNPLUG ELECTRONICS
Your TV, computer and other appliances are constantly sucking away electricity, even if they aren't turned on. Known as standby power, it accounts for 5 to 10 percent of residential energy use, costing the average U.S. household about $100 a year, according to the U.S. Department of Energy. Use a power switch to turn off devices, or unplug ones you're not using, and you'll help save an estimated 44 billion tons of carbon dioxide in the U.S. alone.

7. PUT IN ENERGY-EFFICIENT WINDOWS
Replace leaky, drafty or old windows with dual- or triple-paned glass. These insulate twice as well as older single-paned glass, which translates to lower heating costs— and less energy consumption.

8. PRINT DOUBLE-SIDED
When it's time to hit "print," scroll down on the menu and opt for the two-sided tab. Printing on both sides of a single sheet of paper cuts paper use in half and helps reduce the pollution generated by paper mills.

9. KEEP A REUSABLE BAG HANDY
Despite recent local and state government measures to curb the use of plastic bags, about 40 percent of consumers don't use reusable bags. Keep a small or zip-pouch bag in your purse or glove compartment so you don't have to ask for plastic.

10. GO MEATLESS ON MONDAYS
Eating one less serving of beef every Monday for a year can save the equivalent amount of emissions produced by driving 348 miles. We've got plenty of great plant-based meal ideas starting on page 140 to make this an easy choice!

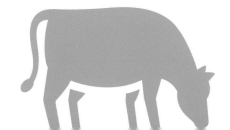

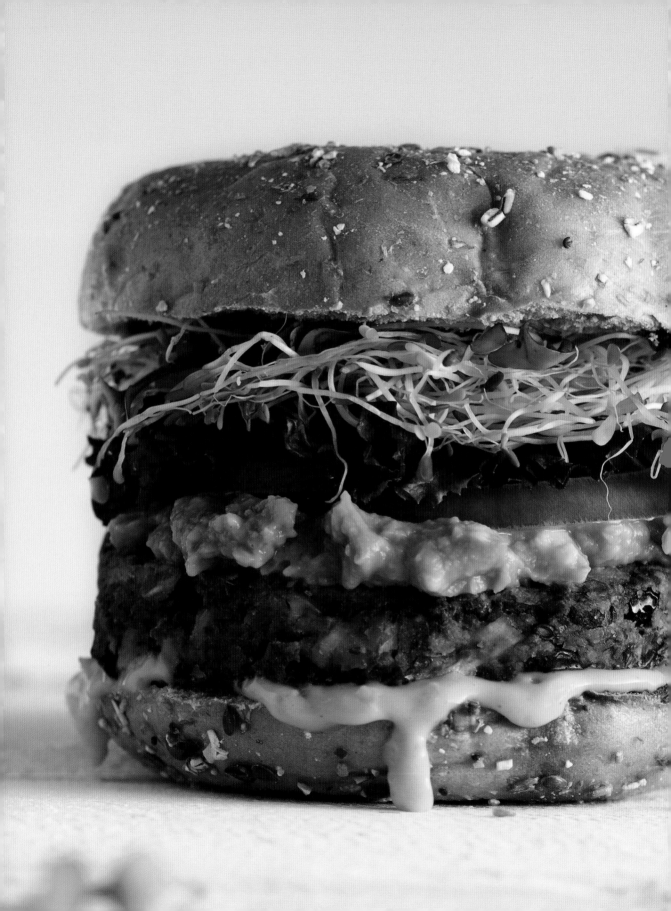

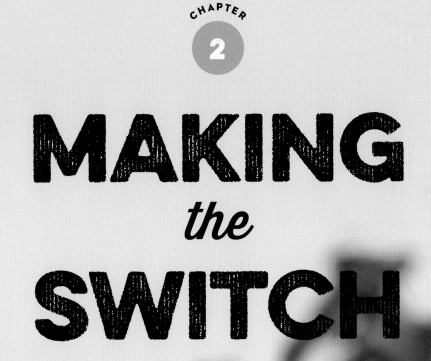

MAKING
the
SWITCH

It's not only easy to boost the amount of plant-based foods in your diet—it's also incredibly delicious! Follow these tips for maximum benefits.

Your Get-Started Guide

Ready to go plant-based?
We tell you everything you need to know about
making the transition, plus tips and tricks for
sticking with your new way of eating. You've got this!

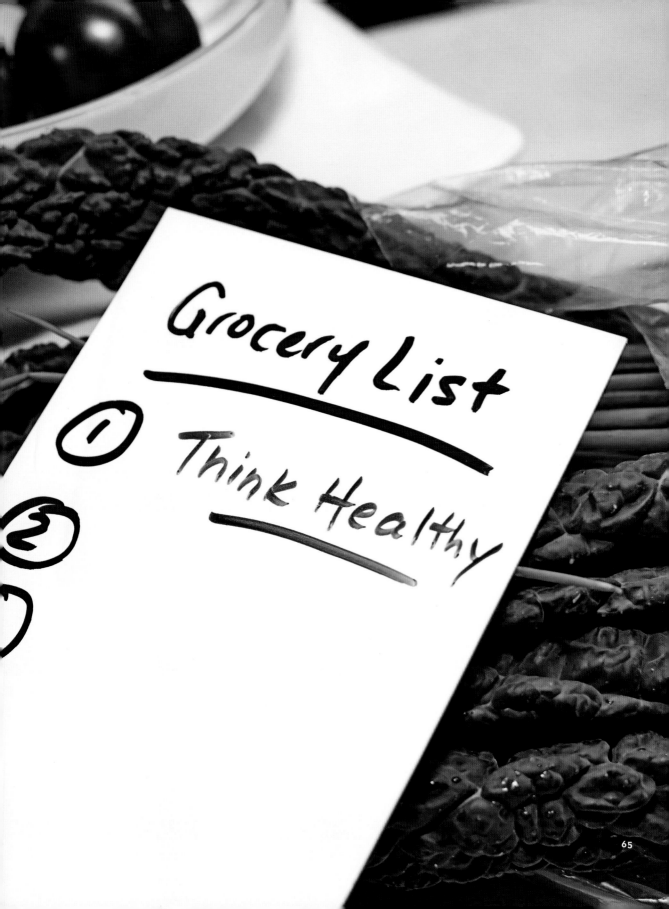

Grocery List

① Think Healthy
②

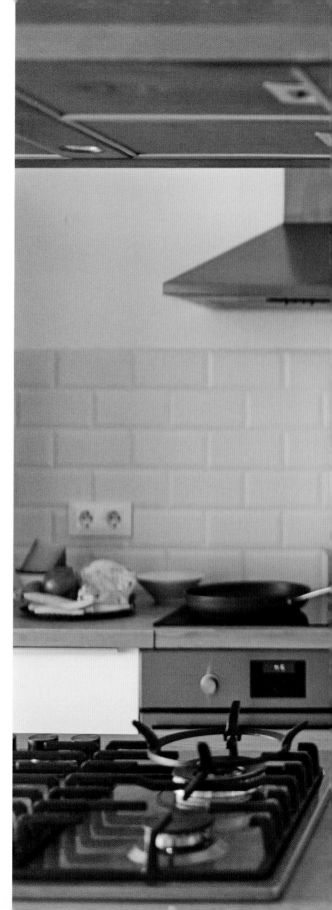

The idea of going plant-based is exciting. Visions of a veggie-packed fridge and overflowing fruit bowls dance in your head, and you can already taste the crisp freshness of the salad and grain bowls that await you. But executing said diet? That's where things can get tricky.

First, there's the actual act of reducing how much meat you eat, which many find easier said than done. Then there's restocking your kitchen, prepping and cooking new meals, and learning how to eat out when meat-centric options may no longer be on the menu. Read on for experts' top 10 tips for making the transition easier, tastier—and fun!

1 Ease Into It

Going plant-based doesn't need to happen overnight. In fact, taking smaller steps to get there may help you adopt long-term changes, says Suzannah Gerber, a plant-based executive chef, cookbook author and food and beverage industry consultant. Try one of these slow-but-steady methods for increasing your plant-based intake and cutting back on meat and other nonplant–based foods.

TRY A TIERED APPROACH
Gerber suggests that people start by cutting out everything that comes from a cow (beef and dairy). Then, when you feel ready, eliminate meat from all animals, followed by cutting out eggs and fish. Even if you're not going vegan, you could take a similar approach. For example: Start by swapping nut milk for your usual half-and-half. Then add at least one fruit or vegetable to every meal and work your way up to having at least one plant-based meal a day.

PLAY WITH PORTION SIZES
You could serve up a little less meat at dinner and add an extra scoop of carrots,

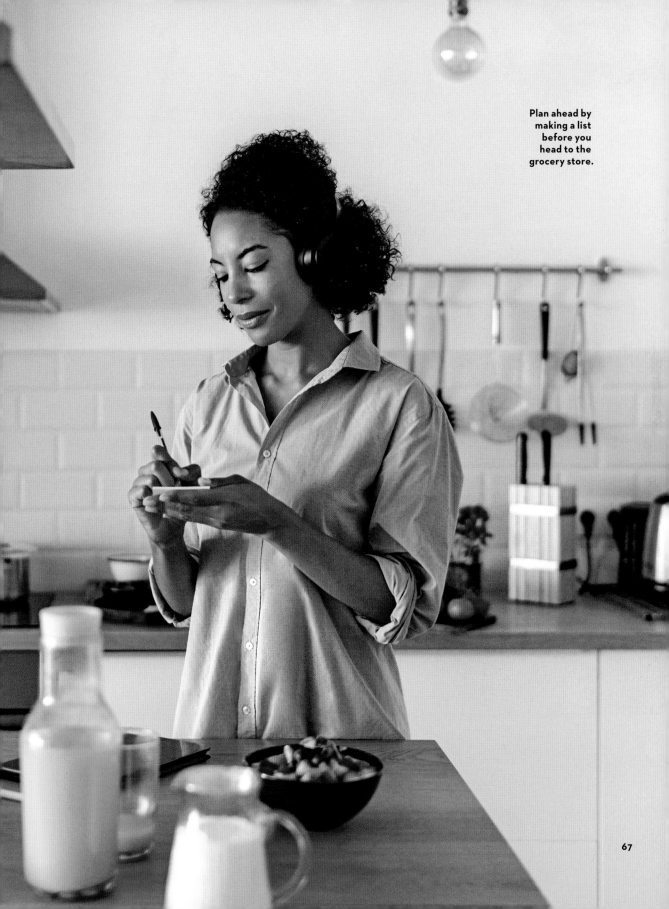

Plan ahead by
making a list
before you
head to the
grocery store.

67

or layer your sandwich with fewer ham slices and more veggie slices. However you choose to go about it, make "More plants!" your motto whenever possible.

ADOPT MEATLESS MONDAYS
One day a week, go meat-free for breakfast, lunch and dinner. Go to meatlessmonday.com to learn more about the movement, get recipe ideas and more.

2 Keep an Open Mind

"Put aside the common myths that you may have heard: that plant-based means a lack of protein, that you'll always be hungry, that it's expensive.... If you're going to try it, commit to doing so with an open mind," says Mamta Valderrama, a vegan educator and blogger at ohforplantsake.com, who has been plant-based for 35 years. As with any lifestyle change, your experience will be unique, so don't let other people's stories and scare tactics ("my cousin became anemic from going vegetarian...") sway you.

3 Plan Ahead

Avoid "I don't know what to eat" moments by taking the time to research recipes for every meal including snacks, drinks and dessert, suggests Valderrama. "Save them to your phone, email them to yourself, print them—be intentional and thoughtful about organizing your recipes to make life easier for yourself." Not sure where to start? Search for recipes that use ingredients you already like. For example, if you can't get enough of asparagus, Google "plant-based asparagus recipes."

4 Manage Your Expectations

Plant-based burgers, chicken fingers, cheese—oh my! These alternatives give plant-based eaters more options than ever, but know that they aren't going to taste like the meat- or dairy-based versions of the foods—and that's OK! "Different doesn't mean bad," says Valderrama. "Plant-based pizza is delicious, but it's different."

5 Set Yourself Up for Cooking Success

You don't need to completely restock your kitchen, but a few key pieces will make plant-based cooking easier. Here's what to get:

GOOD KNIVES You'll be chopping, peeling, dicing and slicing, so make sure you have a set of sharp knives that get the job done. On the must-have list are an all-purpose chef's knife (usually about 8 inches long), a paring knife (3 to 4 inches long) and a serrated knife.

A LARGE CUTTING BOARD Speaking of all that slicing and dicing...you'll want to equip your kitchen with a chopping board that provides ample meal-prepping space. To avoid messes, find an oversize board with nonslip edges to keep it in place and a grooved side to stop juices from running onto the counter.

A POWERFUL BLENDER From smoothies to soups, a dependable blender makes prepping food easier and faster. Consider how big of a model you may need, and features like speed and power. Models with between three and 10 speed settings offer control over what you are chopping. You'll want at least 500 watts of power to make those creamy smoothies.

6 When in Doubt, Add Quinoa

The grain is an excellent protein source for those on a plant-based diet (it's known as a "complete protein" because it contains all nine of the essential amino acids). "It doesn't have much taste on its own, so it can be flavored and

One cup of cooked quinoa has 8 grams of protein and 5 grams of fiber.

SMOOTHIES
MAKE FOR A FAST
AND EASY
PLANT-POWERED
BREAKFAST.

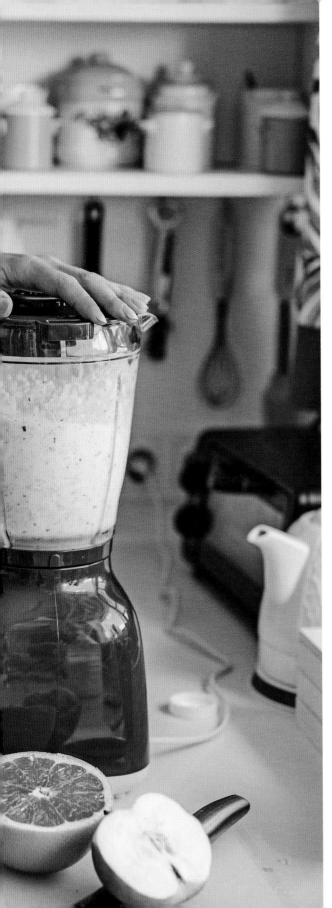

seasoned a million different ways for breakfast, lunch, dinner, salads and snacks," says Valderrama. You could use it in place of oats for a morning breakfast, toss it in a salad at lunch, and put it in a veggie-and-tofu stir-fry at dinner, for example. Make a batch at the start of the week (it only takes about 15 minutes to cook) and store in the fridge for up to four days.

7 Own Your New Way of Eating

Go ahead and get loud about the fact that you're following a plant-based diet—or at least make sure your crew knows that you've changed your way of eating. "Eating plant-based might feel like a challenge in social settings or with family," says Valderrama. "Speak confidently, be clear about what you will or won't eat, and offer to make a dish or share recipes. If you do that, your friends and family will be more likely to support you." Who knows —they may even join you.

8 Ask and You May Receive

These days, more and more restaurants accommodate plant-based eaters, says Gerber. But if there isn't a plant-based entree on the menu, don't panic. Check out the sides served with other dishes and create your own plate. For example, you could have mashed potatoes, broccoli and a portobello "burger"—or ask for roasted veggies in a wrap. (Bonus: These mix-and-match meals are often cheaper, too!)

9 Dodge Tummy Trouble

Plant-based diets tend to be high in fiber. That's great for your health, but increasing your intake too quickly can lead to uncomfortable gas,

bloating and cramping. Avoid stomach issues by following these two tips:

GO GRADUALLY Slowly increase the amount and servings of fruits, vegetables, whole grains and beans you eat—ideally over the course of a few weeks. This gives the bacteria in your digestive system time to adjust to the change.

SIP ON WATER The fluid helps fiber pass smoothly through your digestive system, reducing the chance of constipation or nausea. Aim to drink a glass of water with each meal.

10 Let Your Keyboard Do the Shopping

One brilliant way to make the start of your plant-based journey even easier: Take grocery shopping off your to-do list. Online grocery services have skyrocketed in popularity thanks to the coronavirus pandemic that kept many consumers from wanting to venture into crowded stores. But these services have also gained many fans for their time-saving convenience and hassle-free way of stocking the pantry. A few tips to keep in mind:

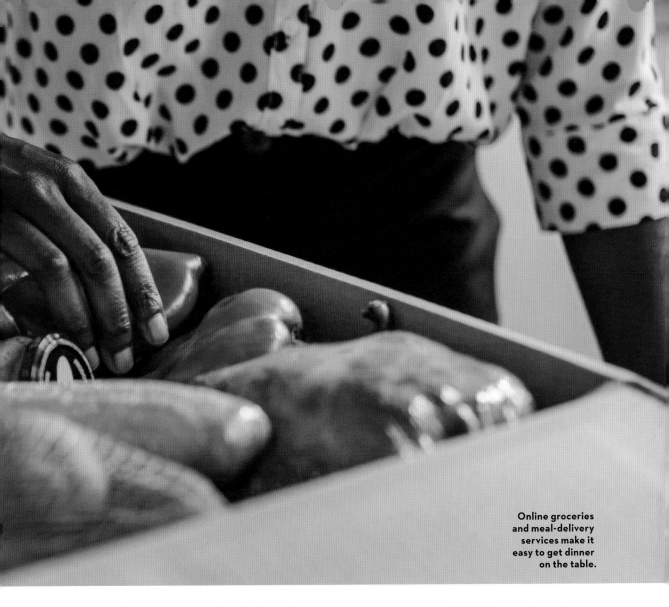

Online groceries and meal-delivery services make it easy to get dinner on the table.

WATCH FOR HIDDEN FEES There's bound to be a price for that convenience. Some online grocers charge a fee for each delivery, others have an unlimited plan with set subscription costs.

DON'T DELAY Just like the stores, orders are first come, first served, so if your cupboard is looking a bit bare, you may want to log on fast and find a delivery spot with a convenient time. Some apps and stores only let you place an order up to 24 hours in advance; others let you schedule regular times for each week or monthly delivery.

KNOW WHAT YOU WANT Since you're not physically browsing the aisles picking up ingredients that might inspire your meals, make a list of what you plan to prepare, including all the necessary ingredients.

CHOOSE REPLACEMENTS If you're using a service like Instacart, where a shopper is doing the picking and choosing for you, you may need more options if your desired items are no longer in stock. It can help to preselect replacement options, or opt out of substitutions altogether if you don't want to take a chance.

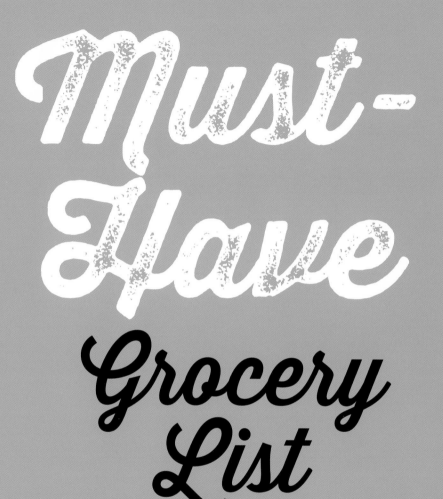

Must-Have Grocery List

Adopting a plant-based diet may mean adding new-to-you produce, grains and other whole foods to your shopping basket. To get you started, we rounded up 14 delicious options along with brilliant, time-saving prepping and cooking tips.

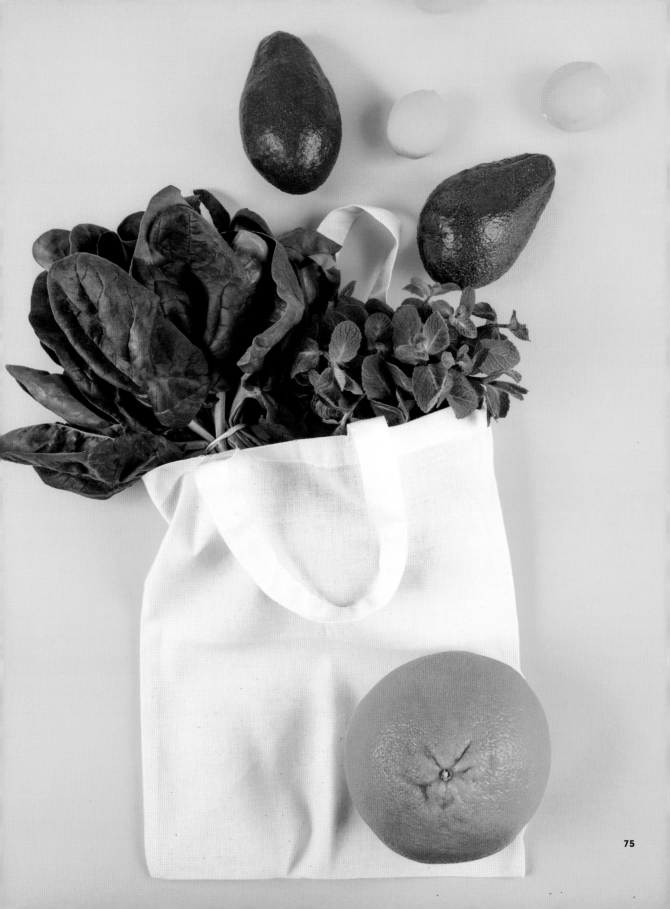

Asparagus

The green version of the veggie, which is in season in the spring, is the most readily available, but asparagus also comes in both a white hue and a pretty purple color, which tends to have a slightly sweeter taste.

THE BENEFITS The willowy vegetable is packed with nutrition: One serving of about five large spears contains 15 percent of the daily recommended amount of vitamin A and 9 percent of vitamin C. It's also high in iron and chromium.

QUICK RECIPE For a simple, speedy side dish, heat the oven to 425°F. Trim asparagus by cutting or snapping off the tougher ends. Arrange spears on a baking sheet and drizzle with olive oil and a squeeze of lemon juice, then season with salt and pepper. Toss to coat, and roast until slightly crispy—about 10 to 20 minutes, depending on how thick the asparagus is.

Avocado

Eating the fruit (yep, avocado is a fruit!) is a great way to work healthy fats into your diet. There are many different varieties, but you're most likely to find Hass avocados in your local supermarket.

THE BENEFITS Avocados contain monounsaturated fat, the "good" type of fat that may help reduce high cholesterol and lower the risk of heart disease and stroke. That healthy fat can also help you feel fuller longer after meals. It's also high in fiber, with 13 grams in one avocado.

HOW TO PICK 'EM A ripe avocado should feel firm but give slightly to light pressure if you squeeze it (gently!) in your palm. If you want to speed up the ripening process of a hard avocado, place it in a paper bag at room temperature. Adding apples or kiwis to the bag can help move along how quickly the avocado ripens.

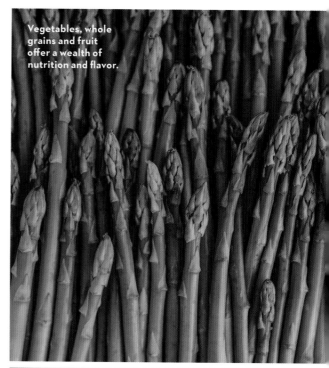

Vegetables, whole grains and fruit offer a wealth of nutrition and flavor.

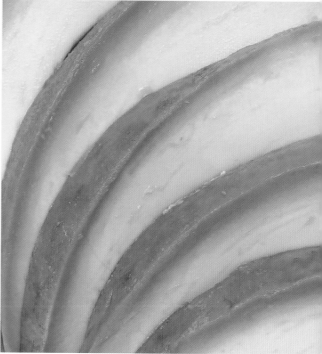

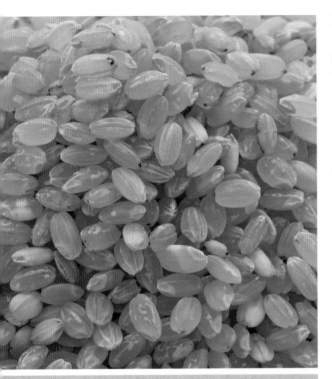

Brown Rice

Unlike white rice, brown rice is a whole grain, meaning that it contains all parts of the grain (only the inedible outer hull is removed). With white rice, other outer layers, called the bran and germ, are also removed, a process that lowers the nutritional value of the rice, including its fiber, vitamins and minerals.

THE BENEFITS Brown rice's bran and germ are high in fiber as well as important vitamins and minerals (such as magnesium and vitamins B1 and B6). Research has even found that substituting brown rice for white could help lower the risk of Type 2 diabetes.

COOKING MUST-KNOW Brown rice can be used in almost any dish in place of white rice, and is a great base for grain bowls. To make perfectly fluffy, delicious brown rice, be sure to rinse it well before cooking. Then, after it's finished cooking, remove from the heat and keep the lid on for at least 10 minutes.

Butternut Squash

The winter squash has a nutty, sweet taste, and is highly versatile, whether used as a substitute for pasta or served up as soup.

THE BENEFITS An excellent source of vitamins and minerals, a serving of butternut squash contains about 300 percent of the recommended daily amount (RDA) of vitamin A and about 50 percent of the RDA of vitamin C. Plus, that bright-orange hue means it's also rich in carotenoids, the disease-fighting phytochemical.

EASY-PEEL TIP The skin on butternut squash can be tough, but this cooking hack makes it easier to remove: Cut off both ends of the squash, then use a fork to prick the squash all over. Microwave for about three to four minutes to soften the skin, and then peel. Try it roasted, steamed, spiralized or mashed, or add to sauces to make them creamier.

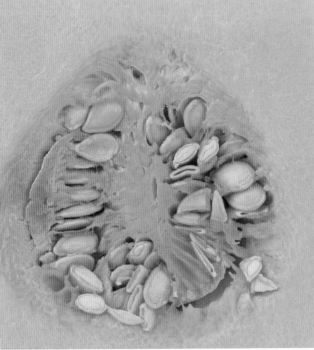

Cauliflower

The award for the most versatile veggie goes to...cauliflower. It's used to make everything from plant-based pizza crusts to "rice," which makes us wonder—is there anything that cauliflower *can't* do?

THE BENEFITS One cup of chopped cauliflower florets contains a whopping 85 percent of the RDA of vitamin C. The low-calorie vegetable is also a good source of folate, a vitamin that's especially important for women who are pregnant, or planning to become pregnant.

WHAT TO LOOK FOR Pick a head of cauliflower that's tightly packed and has bright-green leaves. Once home, transfer the cauliflower to a loosely sealed bag and place a paper towel inside the bag to absorb moisture. This will help extend the life of the veggie. And don't worry too much if some brown spots develop—the discoloration is typically due to oxidation. You can just scrape or cut it away.

Farro

The ancient grain is similar to brown rice, but has a chewier consistency and nuttier flavor.

THE BENEFITS Just a quarter-cup of whole-grain farro has about 7 grams of fiber—about four times as much as brown rice—as well as 7 grams of protein.

HOW TO USE IT As a risotto base, toss it into soups, or sprinkle on top of salads in place of croutons. You can also season farro with salt, pepper and your favorite spices, and serve alone as a side dish.

Kale

Thanks to a spike in kale's popularity, it's easier than ever to find the vegetable in the produce section. Look out for the most common variety, curly kale, as well as others like hearty dinosaur kale (also known as Tuscan kale) and purple-hued redbor kale.

THE BENEFITS Just one cup of chopped kale contains all of your daily recommended vitamins A, C and K—and then some. The veggie is also a great source of potassium and calcium, and is rich in fiber and detoxifying antioxidants.

QUICK SNACK TIP To make deliciously snackable kale chips, preheat the oven to 275°F. Remove kale leaves from stems and chop the leaves into 1- to 2-inch pieces. Toss with olive oil and salt and arrange on a baking tray. Bake until crispy, about 20 minutes, turning the leaves over about halfway through cooking.

Lentils

Depending on where you shop, you may find a number of varieties of this legume on store shelves. Lentils are available in green, brown, black and other colors, and may be sold whole or split.

THE BENEFITS High in both protein and fiber, lentils are a great way to fill up on a plant-based diet. And research has found that eating lentils may help people with diabetes improve their cholesterol levels, and also lowers the risk of breast cancer in women.

SUBSTITUTE Thanks to their meaty texture, lentils are excellent for bulking up a recipe. Add cooked lentils to soups, pastas, salads and more. You can even make a "meatloaf" out of lentils.

Quinoa

Pronounced *keen-waa*, this seed is known as a complete protein because it contains all nine essential amino acids (something that the body can't produce on its own). It comes in multiple colors: white, black, red and yellow.

THE BENEFITS In addition to serving up about 8 grams of protein per serving, quinoa is high in fiber and certain minerals, including magnesium.

GIVE THIS
CHALLENGE
A GO: TRY ONE NEW
PLANT-BASED FOOD
EACH WEEK.

SWEET POTATOES CAN ALSO COME IN WHITE, RED, PINK OR PURPLE.

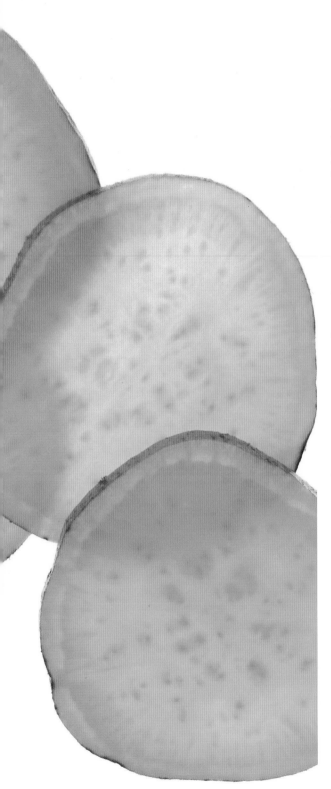

HOW TO USE IT For an easy stove-top breakfast, cook quinoa as you usually would, but substitute almond milk for the water. Add a sweetener (like maple syrup) and some fruit (either frozen or fresh) for a healthy, yummy alternative to oatmeal!

Summer Squash

Zucchini and yellow squash can be eaten raw or cooked. Like cauliflower, squashes can be used in multiple ways: Spiralized zucchini can be used as "pasta," while breaded and baked zucchini sticks can be turned into crispy, yummy "fries."

THE BENEFITS Summer squash has nutrition that spans categories, from vitamins like C and B6 to minerals like potassium, magnesium and copper, as well as antioxidants like carotenoids, plus fiber and protein. And it has all of this nutritional punch with very few calories (about 33 calories in one medium zucchini or yellow squash).

SIMPLE SAUTÉ There are endless ways to cook squash, but for a simple side dish, sauté thinly sliced rounds in olive oil until tender, about 5 minutes, then season.

Sweet Potato

True to its name, the root vegetable has a sweet flavor and bright-orange flesh.

THE BENEFITS Sweet potatoes are sky-high in vitamin A in the form of beta-carotene, an antioxidant that boosts the health of the skin, eyes and immune system. They're also a good source of filling fiber.

HEALTH HACK To get the most beta-carotene benefits, boil your sweet potatoes. This method retains more of the nutrients than baking or frying. To make mashed sweet potatoes, boil rinsed and cubed sweet potatoes for about 20 minutes, or until tender when pierced with a fork. Add a small amount of plant-based butter and milk, and mash.

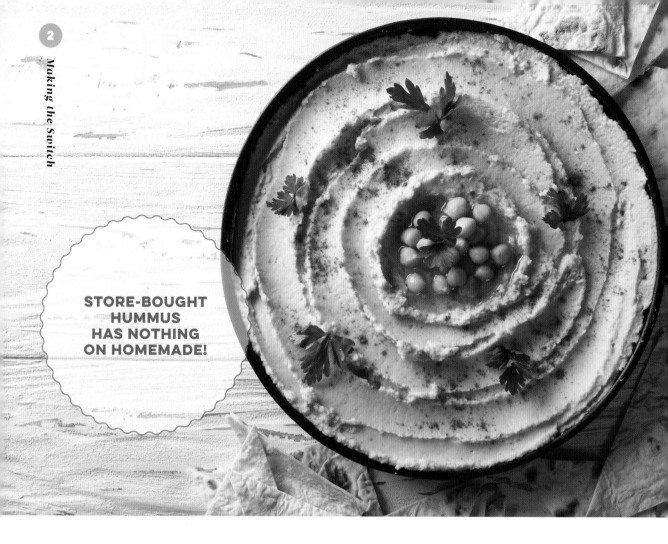

STORE-BOUGHT
HUMMUS
HAS NOTHING
ON HOMEMADE!

Tahini

Made from sesame seeds, tahini is a main ingredient in hummus. But you can also try the creamy condiment as a dip for raw veggies, a spread on toast or salad dressing.

THE BENEFITS Tahini is a good source of protein, calcium and iron, and it also contains heart-healthy monounsaturated fat.

EASY HUMMUS RECIPE For a quick, better-than-store-bought hummus, combine 1 can rinsed chickpeas, 2 tablespoons tahini, ¼ cup olive oil, 1 garlic clove and a big squeeze of lemon juice in a food processor. Purée until smooth (add water if needed to thin the hummus out). Serve topped with a drizzle of olive oil and a sprinkle of paprika.

Tempeh

To make tempeh, soybeans are cooked and fermented and then formed into a dense, nutty-tasting cake that tends to absorb the flavors of whatever else it's cooked with. Because it holds its shape well when cooked, it makes a fantastic meat replacement in recipes like tacos and stir-fries.

THE BENEFITS *Hello*, protein! One 3-ounce serving of tempeh provides 16 grams of the macronutrient.

HOW TO CUT IT According to America's Test Kitchen, tempeh cooks best when it is cut into slabs about ⅜-inch thick. This will allow for a crispy edge to form when it is seared in a pan.

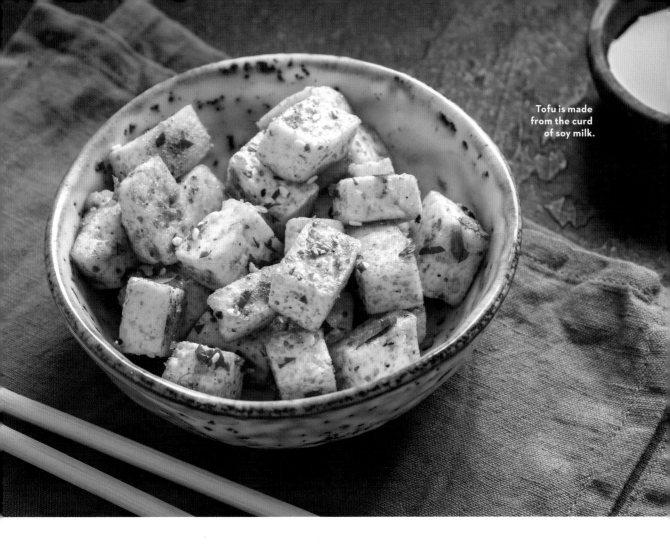

Tofu is made from the curd of soy milk.

Tofu

Also known as bean curd, tofu is made from coagulated soy milk. It comes in several firmness levels, depending on how much of the liquid has been pressed out. Options range from silken, which has a custard-esque texture and is great in smoothies and desserts, to extra firm, which can be sliced, cubed and grilled.

THE BENEFITS You might remember concerns about whether a diet rich in soy could increase the risk of breast cancer, but don't let that scare you away from tofu. According to the Mayo Clinic, we now know that eating soy foods over the course of a lifetime may actually reduce the risk of breast cancer in women, and that moderate amounts (one to two servings a day) won't increase the risk.

PREP TIP Pressing firm and extra-firm tofu before cooking helps to release water, reducing the chance that the tofu will fall apart or crumble while cooking it. To press your tofu, sandwich the block between clean kitchen towels (or folded paper towels). Place a cutting board on top of the top towel and put a weight—like a heavy book or pot—on top of the cutting board. Let sit for 20 to 30 minutes (replace the towels halfway through if they become too wet), and then cook as desired. You can also speed things up with a tofu press.

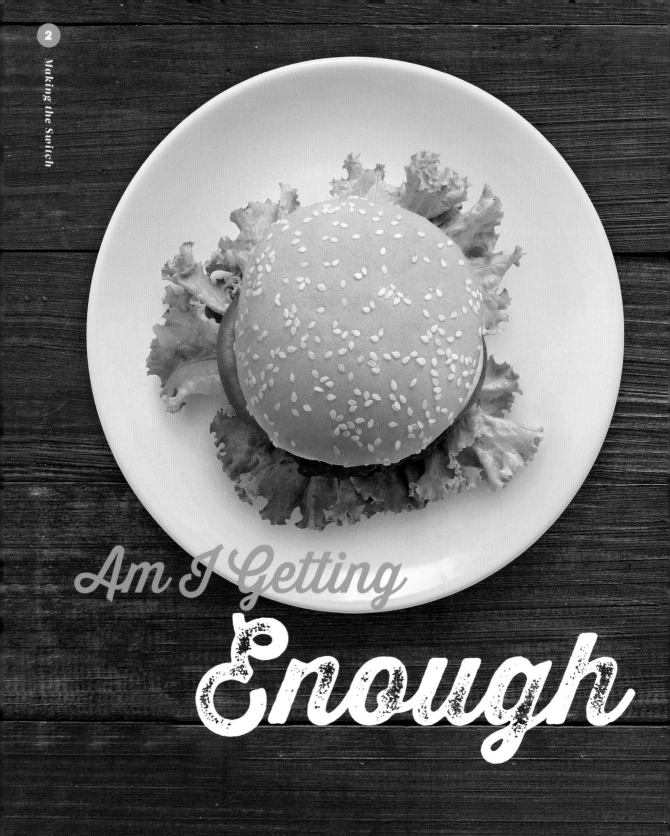

Am I Getting Enough

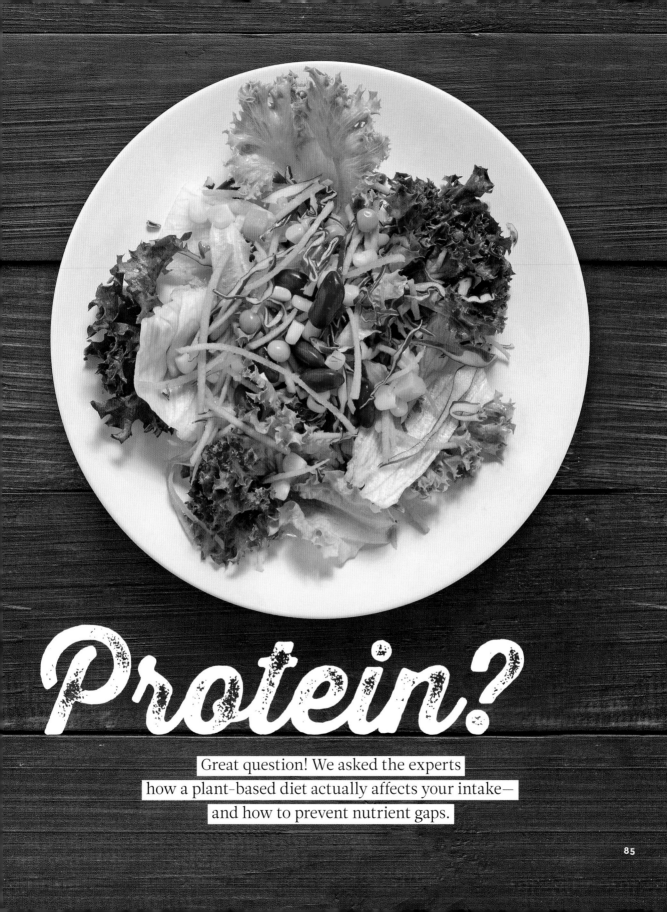

Protein?

Great question! We asked the experts
how a plant-based diet actually affects your intake—
and how to prevent nutrient gaps.

Thinking about adopting a plant-based lifestyle? Prepare to become familiar with the question from concerned friends that will be repeated like a broken record: *How do you get your protein?*

Many people assume that giving up meat means missing out on protein. Not true! In fact, research shows that most vegetarians and vegans meet and even exceed their protein requirements, according to the Academy of Nutrition and Dietetics. And you don't have to chug protein shakes all day long to make that happen.

"Protein is in pretty much every food we eat—even in fruits and vegetables," says Jennifer Mimkha, MPH, a plant-based registered dietitian at Prana Nutrition in Tampa, Florida. "If you're getting enough calories in your diet, then you typically are getting enough protein."

So why are we so quick to question whether a plant-based diet has enough protein? Most people aren't clear on how much protein we *should* be getting. Americans consume more protein than people in any other country do, so we have a skewed view of what's "normal." "People think we need more protein than we do," says Betsy Redmond, PhD, a registered dietitian in Atlanta.

That said, your family and friends may be on to something. People who eat less meat *do* generally get less protein—but that's not bad. "This may be part of the benefit of going plant-based, since excess protein can have negative health issues," says Redmond.

The "right" amount of protein can look different for different people, but dietitians generally recommend that plant-based eaters consume 1 gram per every kilogram of body weight. If you're a 140-pound woman, that translates into approximately 64 grams of protein a day. (Read "Packed With Protein," opposite page, to see how you can meet those needs by layering your meals with a variety of high-protein foods.)

And here's some good news: There's no need to start micromanaging your protein intake by tallying up how much you're getting at each and every meal. Instead, focus on filling your plate with a variety of real, whole foods.

"Rather than worrying about protein when planning meals, I encourage people to consider the nutrient density of foods they are about to consume, choosing foods filled with fiber, antioxidants, vitamins, minerals and water," says Mimkha. If you're checking off all of those boxes, you're most likely getting a healthy amount of protein.

A Day Full of Protein (and Other Important Nutrients!)

HERE'S HOW YOU CAN MEET YOUR GOAL, FROM BREAKFAST TO BEDTIME.

BREAKFAST
Make plant-based oatmeal by cooking whole oats with soy milk, berries, peanut butter, and hemp seeds, flaxseeds and chia seeds. Sprinkle with cinnamon, walnuts and pumpkin seeds.

LUNCH
Prepare a plant-based power bowl by layering spinach and kale with garbanzo beans, farro, tofu, sunflower seeds and hummus. Toss in any other veggies you have in the fridge!

DINNER
Whip up a homemade black bean–quinoa burger sprinkled with nutritional yeast. Top your veggie burger with tomato, onion and avocado slices, and serve with a side of peas.

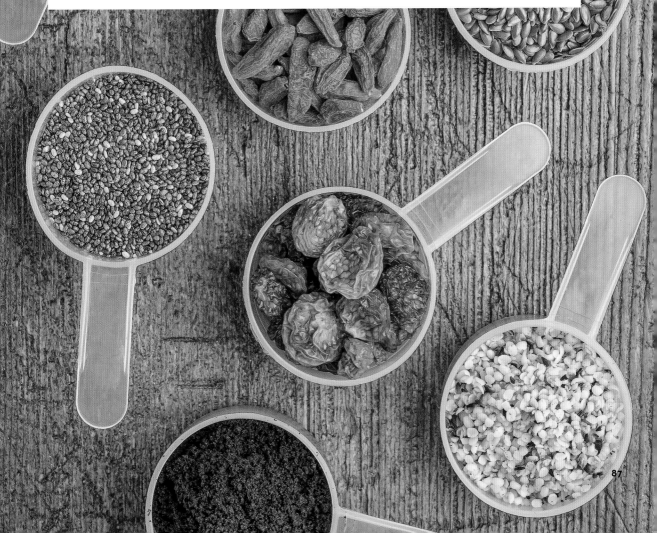

PACKED WITH PROTEIN

WORK THESE FOODS CONTAINING HIGH AMOUNTS OF THE NUTRIENT INTO YOUR DIET.

LENTILS
18 g per 1 cup

EDAMAME
18 g per 1 cup

**BLACK, KIDNEY
AND PINTO BEANS**
16 g per 1 cup

TEMPEH
16 g per ½ cup

CHICKPEAS
14 g per 1 cup

QUINOA
12 g per ½ cup

HEMP SEEDS
10 g per
3 tablespoons

TOFU
10 g per ½ cup

PUMPKIN SEEDS
9 g per ¼ cup

AMARANTH
9 g per 1 cup

PEANUT BUTTER
8 g per 2 tablespoons

SOY MILK
8 g per 1 cup

PEAS, COOKED
8 g per 1 cup

ALMONDS
6 g per ¼ cup

PISTACHIOS
6 g per ¼ cup

WHEAT BERRIES
6 g per ½ cup

SUNFLOWER SEEDS
6 g per ¼ cup

KAMUT
6 g per ½ cup

CHIA SEEDS
5 g per 3 tablespoons

OATS
5 g per ½ cup

SPINACH, COOKED
5 g per 1 cup

BROCCOLI
5 g per 2 cups

WHAT YOU NEED TO KNOW ABOUT VITAMINS AND MINERALS

The average American diet is low in vitamins A, C, D, E and folate; calcium, magnesium, fiber and potassium, according to findings from the 2015 Dietary Guidelines Advisory Committee. While heavy meat-eaters tend to consume the lowest amounts of these nutrients, simply cutting meat from your diet won't guarantee you've covered all your nutritional bases. The best way to ensure that you don't have any nutrient gaps is to focus your plant-based efforts on a varied diet.

How can you make sure it's varied? Eat foods from every color of the rainbow—every day. To keep yourself on track, download the free Daily Dozen app from Michael Greger, MD, author of *How Not to Die*. It has a daily checklist so you can prevent nutrition holes from sabotaging your health.

It's also a good idea to check in with a dietitian or doctor. They can use a blood test to measure whether you have specific deficiencies. While most plant-based eaters choosing a varied diet of whole foods will not have to take any supplements beyond B12 and vitamin D, depending on your individual results, you may find that you need to up certain foods, or boost with a vitamin. Use this cheat sheet to make sure you're including the vitamins and minerals that plant-based eaters (and people in general!) don't always get enough of in their diet.

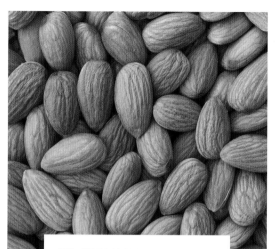

TO GET MORE CALCIUM
EAT soy foods (edamame, tofu and tempeh), beans (winged, white, navy and black), almonds and almond butter, and dark leafy greens

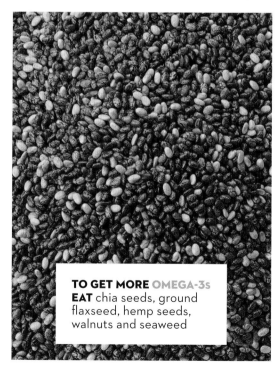

TO GET MORE OMEGA-3s
EAT chia seeds, ground flaxseed, hemp seeds, walnuts and seaweed

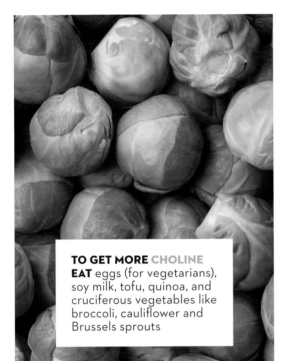

TO GET MORE CHOLINE
EAT eggs (for vegetarians), soy milk, tofu, quinoa, and cruciferous vegetables like broccoli, cauliflower and Brussels sprouts

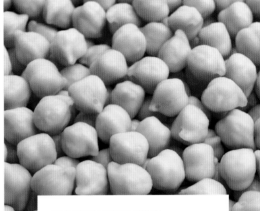

TO GET MORE IRON
EAT pumpkin seeds, kale, lentils, chickpeas, beans, tofu, cashews, chia seeds, flaxseeds and hemp seeds, dried apricots and figs, raisins, quinoa, and fortified breakfast cereals

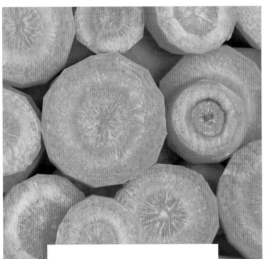

TO GET MORE VITAMIN A
EAT carrots, butternut squash, sweet potato, dried apricots, spinach and cantaloupe

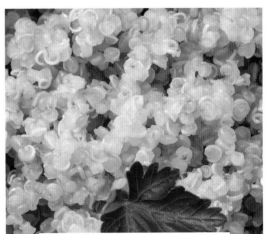

TO GET MORE ZINC
EAT beans, chickpeas, lentils, tofu, walnuts, cashews, bread, quinoa, chia seeds, flaxseeds, hemp seeds and pumpkin seeds

The ‘C’ Word

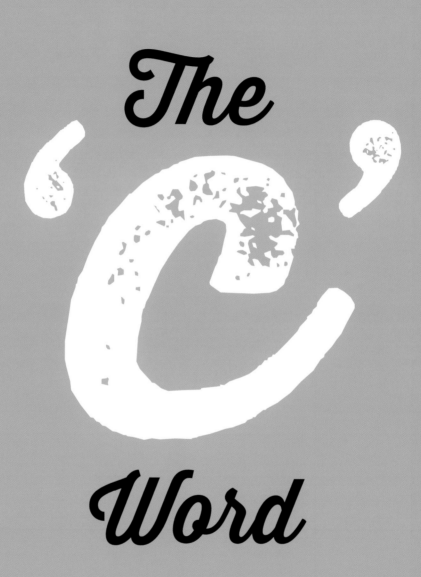

Carbs have a branding problem. Don't let that stop you from enjoying them.

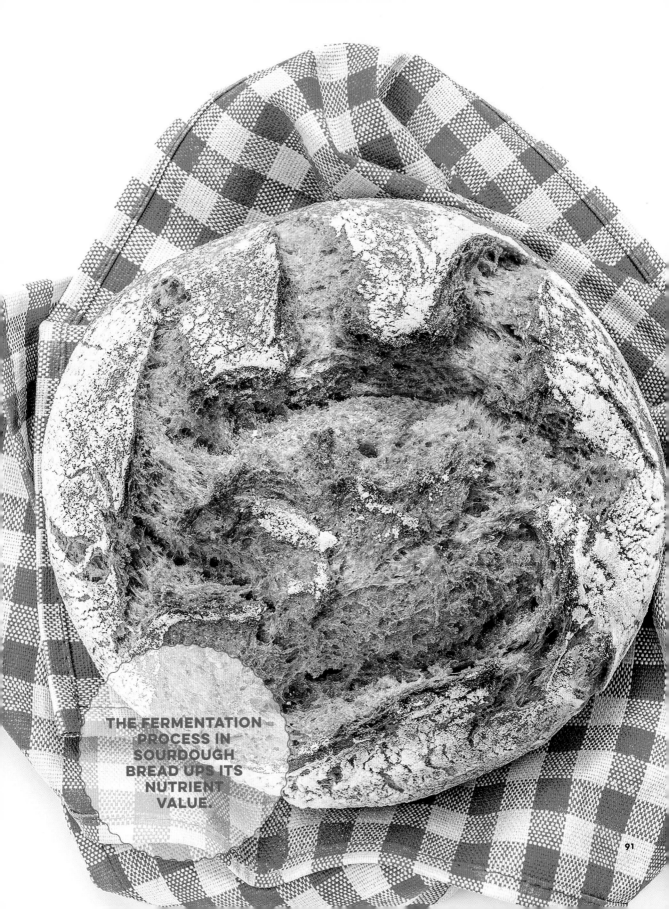

THE FERMENTATION PROCESS IN SOURDOUGH BREAD UPS ITS NUTRIENT VALUE.

Carbohydrates are misunderstood. Back in the '80s and '90s, they reigned supreme, especially when nutrition experts advocated cutting back on fat. People listened—but replaced their fat with refined carbohydrates, which are less healthy than "complex" carbs (some experts believe this spurred an increase in heart disease and obesity). Now, it's carbs that are on the run. Low-carb advocates recommend cutting way back on the crucial macronutrient— it's a pillar of the ketogenic, paleo, Atkins and Zone diets. Then there are those who single out certain foods, such as sugars and bananas, as being "bad" for you.

While some people certainly thrive on low-carb diets, and reducing added sugars *is* beneficial for your health, there's no reason to completely cut carbs out of your diet. "Carbohydrates are the preferred source of fuel for your body," explains Amy Kimberlain, RDN, national spokesperson for the Academy of Nutrition and Dietetics. Still, that doesn't mean you have a free pass to gorge on carbs. Portions always matter, and not all carbs are created equal. Just as there are different grades of gas for your car, there are different types of carbs—some will sustain you, while others will leave you feeling empty. "You want to fuel your body at a higher octane," Kimberlain says. "Yes, there will be days when you have a dessert. That's normal. But if dessert is your primary source of fuel, that will negatively affect how you feel."

High-Octane Fuel

Carbohydrates can be split into two categories—complex and simple—based on their structure. Complex carbs are made of three or more sugars bonded together in long chains, while simple carbs are made of one or two sugars bonded in shorter chains. Carbohydrates can also be divided into starches, fibers and sugars. Starches and fibers are complex carbs, while sugars are simple carbs.

Sources of complex carbs include whole grains, such as 100 percent whole-wheat bread and pasta; brown rice, farro, barley and oats; beans and legumes; potatoes and sweet potatoes; winter squash, such as acorn and butternut; other vegetables; and fruit. Complex carbs are rich in nutrients and are digested more slowly, giving you more sustained energy.

Research links complex carbs with a variety of health benefits. In particular, higher intakes of whole grains may reduce the risk of several diseases. In a series of reviews published in *The Lancet* in 2019, scientists analyzed data from 185 prospective studies and 58 clinical trials. They found that people who consumed the most whole grains had a 13 to 33 percent lower risk of coronary heart disease, stroke, Type 2 diabetes, colorectal cancer and early death compared with people who consumed the least amount of whole grains.

Part of this benefit may be thanks to the fiber in whole grains, which is associated with lower blood pressure, total cholesterol and body weight. "Fiber is the part of the plant that you're not able to digest," Kimberlain explains. "Because soluble fiber slows the absorption of food after a meal and helps moderate the rise and fall of blood glucose, it can help you feel fuller longer." This may lead to eating less and managing weight. (Eating 25 to 29 grams of fiber a day has been linked with the most health benefits.)

Complex carbs also provide vitamins and minerals—and some, such as beans and whole grains, contain protein, making them nature's little nutrient multitaskers.

WHAT
YOU EAT
WITH YOUR
CARBS MAKES
A BIG
DIFFERENCE.

But there's more. Some complex carbs are sources of resistant starch. This type of fiber passes through the small intestine without being digested. When it reaches the large intestine, the fibers ferment and feed gut-friendly bugs, Kimberlain explains. Studies show resistant starch may help you eat less and improve insulin sensitivity, which may reduce the risk of diabetes. Good sources of resistant starch include green bananas, plantains, beans, peas, legumes, oats, and cooked and cooled potatoes and rice.

Low-Octane Carbs

Simple carbs include processed, refined flour, which makes its way into pasta, bread, crackers and other products; white rice; and sugars, including "natural" ones like honey and maple syrup. Your body easily breaks these down, giving you a surge of immediate energy as your blood sugar spikes. But then it typically crashes, along with your stamina. This can also make you feel hungrier sooner than you would if you ate complex carbs with fiber. In addition, simple carbohydrates tend to lack fiber, vitamins and minerals—meaning they're what's called empty calories.

All of this can be detrimental for your health, especially if you're drinking your carbs. For every 12 ounces of sugary beverages such as soda, fruit juice and sports drinks consumed a day, risk of death from any cause increases 11 percent, according to a study published in 2019

in *JAMA Network Open*. Other research published in the *British Medical Journal* found that, for every 3.3 ounces of sugary drinks consumed a day, the risk of cancer increased 18 percent. In both studies, even 100 percent fruit juice had negative effects.

Fuel for Your Best Performance

You don't have to cut out simple carbs completely, but, for your health, it's best to emphasize complex carbs. Kimberlain recommends making at least half of your daily grains whole grains and minimizing processed, refined carbohydrates. The USDA recommends women under 50 get a minimum of 3 "ounce-equivalents" (48 g) of whole grains a day; men should get at least 3 or 4 (48 g to 64 g).

In addition, instead of having a huge plate of pasta at dinner, "divide your carbs throughout your day so you have stable energy," Kimberlain says. Balancing your meals with a mix of carbs, healthy fats, protein and nonstarchy vegetables will also help. Consider cutting back on your pasta portion and top it with chicken or tofu and veggies cooked in a little olive oil.

Aim for variety as well. "When I have grains, I try to rotate things like rice, whole-wheat pasta, farro and barley," Kimberlain says. This way, you not only enjoy a range of flavors as well as vitamins and minerals, you can notice how your body responds to different foods. You may find that millet leaves you more satisfied than brown rice, or that pasta really does give you excellent energy to go running.

Lastly, don't feel pressured to give up the carbs you love. If white rice is part of your culture, enjoy it, perhaps in a smaller portion with a little more black beans. Consuming carbs the healthy way means paying attention to quantity and quality.

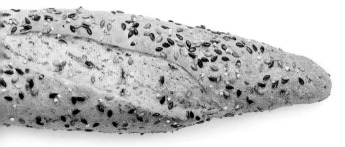

You don't always have to pass on pasta, but keep portions in check.

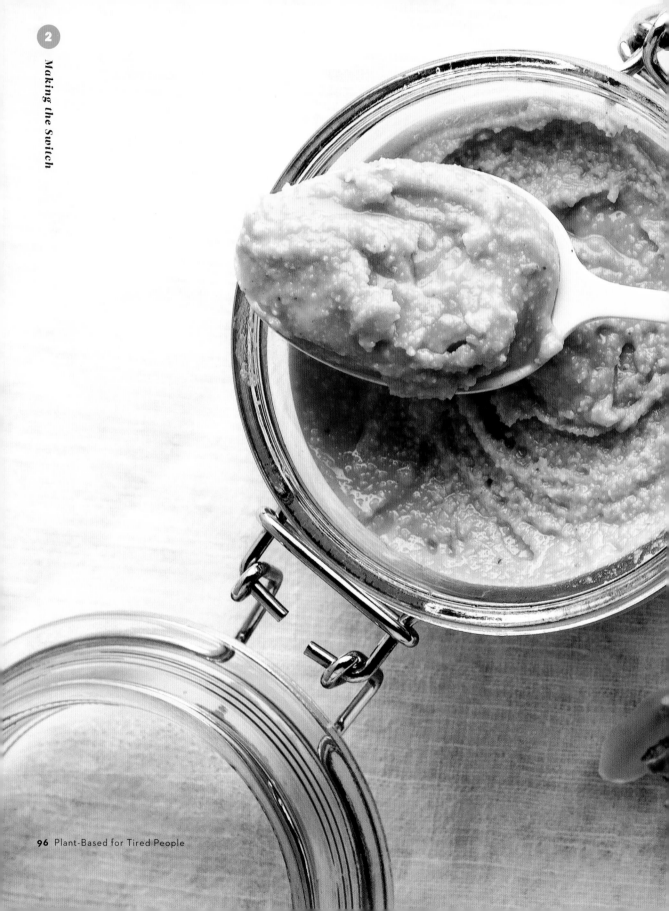

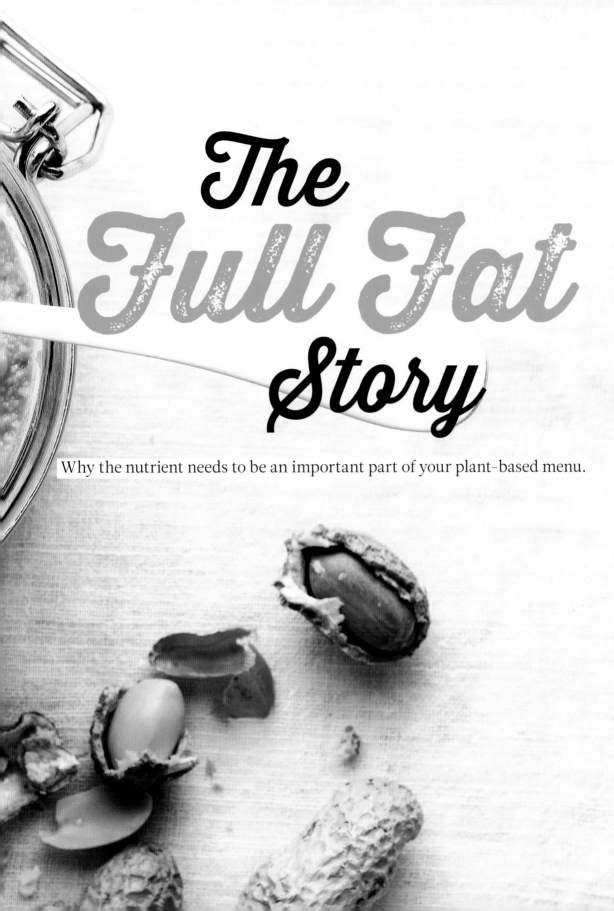

The *Full Fat* Story

Why the nutrient needs to be an important part of your plant-based menu.

nce avoided or at least severely minimized as part of a healthy diet, fat is no longer the bad guy it was made out to be. For decades, this essential macronutrient has been dissed and downgraded, accused of causing ailments like obesity and heart disease. Food labels everywhere once touted "Non-Fat!" and "Reduced Fat!" as selling points. Today, we have a new understanding of fat, but many people remain confused about which kinds are the best to eat—and whether some are still considered unhealthy. Luckily, new research in just the past few years has revealed a lot more about how fat works in the body and which types to choose. Following is a breakdown of the various categories and the bottom line on each.

Saturated Fats

These types of fats, which are solid at room temperature and mostly derived from animal sources (think cheese, butter and whole milk), were long blamed for raising blood cholesterol and contributing to heart disease. But the tide has been turning, says David Ludwig, MD, PhD, a professor of nutrition at the Harvard T.H. Chan School of Public Health. "Saturated fat used to be public-health enemy No. 1," he explains, "but it's neither that, nor exactly a health food. Overall, it's rather neutral, depending on what other foods are eaten with it or substituted for it."

Research is backing that up. A report in *Annals of Internal Medicine* analyzed 76 studies and concluded there was no evidence for avoiding saturated fats in favor of unsaturated. Another meta-analysis, in *The American Journal of Clinical Nutrition*, has found no support for the idea that saturated fat increases the risk of heart disease or stroke. Despite those and similar findings, the American Heart Association still recommends severely limiting saturated fats to 6 percent of total calories per day.

So what gives? Well, it's complicated, says Ludwig. "For instance, saturated fats do somewhat raise LDL, the so-called 'bad' cholesterol. But at the same time, they raise the 'good' HDL cholesterol, which is protective, and they also lower triglycerides." And the higher your HDL, the better. Balance is the key, says Kendra Whitmire, a dietitian in Laguna Beach, California, who practices functional and therapeutic nutrition. "You don't want to eat only saturated fats," she says. "You'll want to balance those with omega-3 fatty acids and other forms. But if you're getting your saturated fat from whole-food sources—butter, cheese, eggs —in addition to some fish oils and vegetable and nut oils, it's not going to be a problem."

Unsaturated Fats

These fats can be found in two forms, monounsaturated and polyunsaturated, and many healthy foods naturally contain some of each. These are the fats you'll hear characterized as "healthy," because in general, they've been shown to raise HDL cholesterol and lower LDL.

Monounsaturated fats are abundant in olives, avocados and many nuts, such as walnuts—and also in their resulting oils when pressed into liquid form. These are generally "good-for-you" fats, especially the heart-healthy, HDL-boosting olive oil, though there are some exceptions.

On the polyunsaturated side, one type, in particular, has been found to be especially beneficial: the now world-famous omega-3 fatty acids, which have come to be seen almost as a kind of wonder fat. In addition to their cardiovascular benefits, omega-3s

Cacao (yes, the kind in chocolate!) has a blend of healthy fats plus antioxidants.

have been found to reduce inflammation in the body, help fight depression and anxiety, lower blood pressure, reduce cancer risk, improve sleep quality and skin health, possibly reduce the risk of dementia, and more. Omega-3s are abundant in fatty fish, like salmon, mackerel and herring, but you can also find them in plant sources such as flaxseeds, chia seeds and walnuts.

But, just to muddy the waters a bit, another form of polyunsaturated fats, omega-6, is a little less golden. This type, which includes many vegetable oils like soybean, corn and safflower, is also essential to health—in moderation. Because these oils are widely used in restaurant and packaged-food preparation and have also benefited from a reputation as heart-healthy and superior to saturated fats, we now consume many more of them than we did a century ago. Here, the devil may be in the dose—or, more precisely, in the ratio.

Humans evolved on a diet with a ratio of omega-6 to omega-3 fatty acids of about 1 to 1, according to many evolutionary and Paleolithic-nutrition studies. But in the typical Western diet today, the ratio is 15 or 16 to 1, a staggering difference that is thought to promote many common ailments, including cardiovascular disease, cancer and autoimmune disorders. Research has shown that lowering the ratio down to 3 or 4 to 1 can help prevent those conditions.

Trans Fats

The fourth category is man-made fats—and here, the answer is simple: Just say no. Trans fats came about when companies in the early 20th century found a way to make liquid fats shelf-stable (useful for packaged goods, like crackers and breads) by transforming them into solid fats through hydrogenation. This processing, though, made them dangerous, and trans fats were ultimately found to increase LDL cholesterol, reduce HDL, create inflammation and cause insulin resistance—all of which greatly raise the risk of heart disease. Trans fats are now banned by the FDA, but are permitted in small amounts, so look at labels for information.

Plant-Based Fat All-Stars

THE FOOD	TYPE	AMOUNT
Avocado	Mostly monounsaturated	15 g/medium size fruit
Cacao Nibs	Saturated and monounsaturated	12 g/1 ounce
Chia Seeds	Mostly polyunsaturated	4 g/1 tablespoon
Edamame	Monounsaturated and polyunsaturated	5 g/cup
Extra-Virgin Olive Oil	Monounsaturated and polyunsaturated	14 g/tablespoon
Flaxseeds	Polyunsaturated (omega-3s)	4 g/1 tablespoon
Olives	Monounsaturated	3 g/ounce
Peanut Butter	Monounsaturated and polyunsaturated	6 g/1 tablespoon
Walnuts	Mostly polyunsaturated (omega-3s)	18 g/1 ounce

COOKING WITH FAT

IT'S AN ESSENTIAL INGREDIENT FOR MANY MEALS, SO MAKE THE MOST OF IT.

AVOCADO OIL
Whole avocados are high in monounsaturated fat as well as a host of other important nutrients—and the oil pressed from the fruit is equally healthful. It's also incredibly versatile when used in cooking, with just about the highest smoke point of any oil—520°F—meaning that you can cook at a very high heat without having it break down, burn or have an effect on taste.

COCONUT OIL
While coconut oil is saturated, it operates differently in your body than animal-based saturated fats. It also may have special benefits: It boosts fat burning and contains medium-chain triglycerides (MCTs), which go straight to the liver to then be used as a quick source of energy.

EXTRA-VIRGIN OLIVE OIL
The benefits of this mainly monounsaturated fat are many: It is antioxidant, anti-inflammatory and anti-bacterial; it protects against heart disease; and it raises HDL cholesterol. It has a medium smoke point (the heat at which an oil starts to degrade), so it's fine for sautéing but not for cooking at very high temperatures. It excels in sauces and salad dressings.

SESAME OIL
Sesame seeds have been pressed to extract their oils for thousands of years. They bring a distinctive flavor, particularly in savory Asian-inspired dishes, along with a hefty amount of omega-3s and compounds called phytosterols that reduce cholesterol uptake in the body.

WALNUT OIL
Walnuts are a highly versatile nut, and so is the oil they provide—which is rich in omega-3 fatty acids as well as vitamins like manganese, niacin, potassium and zinc. However, walnut oil does not cook well at high heat, so its rich, nutty flavor is better served as a star ingredient in sauces, salad dressings or in toppings for grilled vegetables.

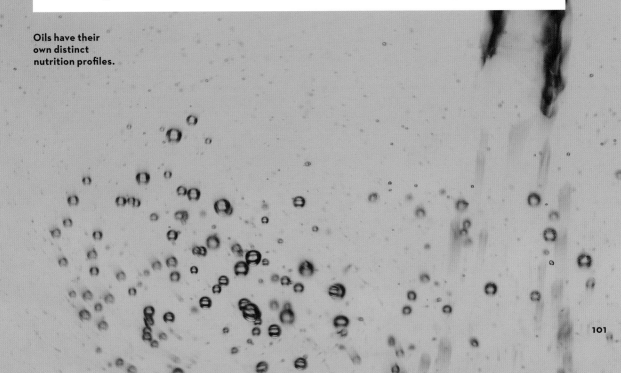

Oils have their own distinct nutrition profiles.

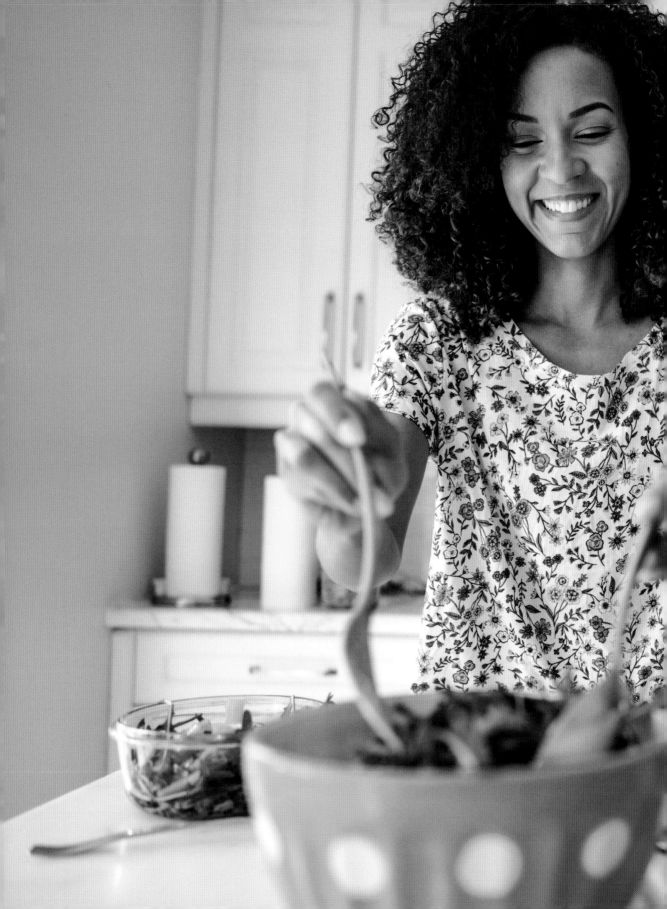

CHAPTER

3

SMART LIVING

Made the decision to keep plants front and center on your plate? Congrats! Now here's how to make it an easy fit in your daily routine.

The Fake-Meat Boom

Once considered "crunchy" and far from mainstream, plant-based eating is now taking over the wellness world —and food companies are taking note, developing meat alternatives that taste more like the real thing than ever before.

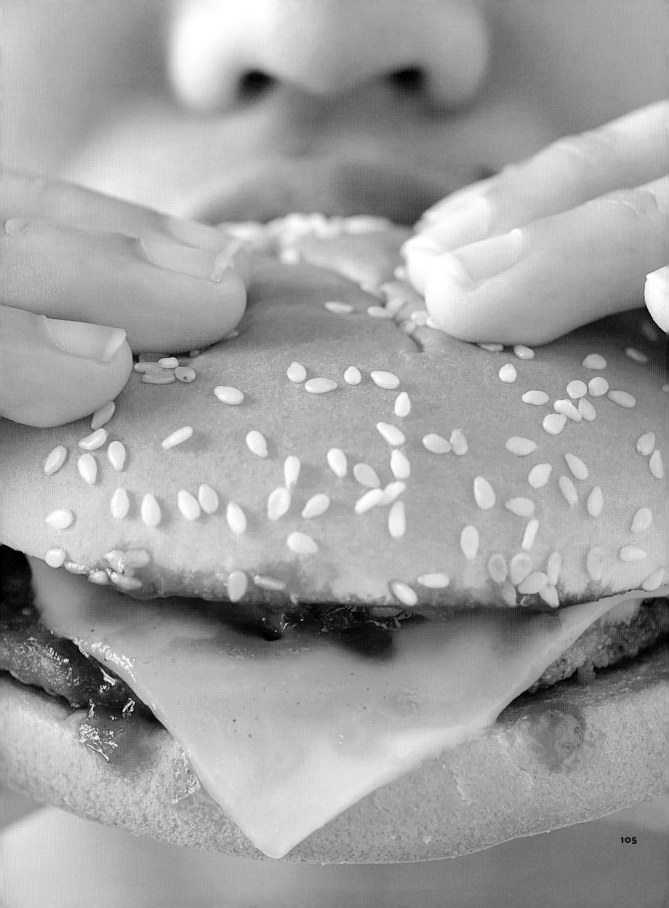

f you strolled a supermarket's frozen-foods section just 10 years ago, you may have come across a few plant-based veggie burgers, but the selection would have likely stopped there. And if you had asked for plant-based options at a restaurant, there's a good chance you would have been pointed to a less-than-appetizing side salad.

Today, those same aisles are packed with faux-meat burgers as well as plant-based "nuggets," "meatballs" and more. Restaurants are also jumping on the growing trend with mouthwatering meat alternatives.

Numbers tell the same story: The plant-based food and beverage industry—including faux, plant-based meats—is officially booming. In 2019, the plant-based-foods retail market was worth $4.5 billion, an 11 percent increase from 2018, according to The Good Food Institute and the Plant Based Foods Association, and research shows that it's expected to keep climbing. Even companies that traditionally sell animal products, like Tyson Foods, are diving into the fake-meat business, and the ever-popular Trader Joe's grocery chain recently came out with its own plant-based burger.

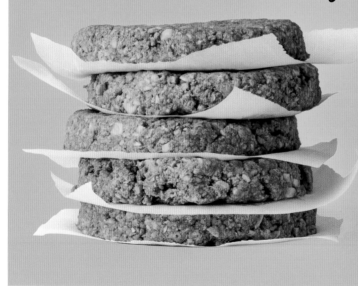

Some veggie burgers are fortified with vitamin B12 and zinc.

Are Plant-Based Burgers Healthy?

That depends. "Just because something is a plant-based food, that doesn't mean it's necessarily healthy," says Michael Smith, MD, senior medical director at WebMD. "You still should pay attention to labels and ensure that they're supporting your overall health goals." Certain meat-alternative burgers, for example, have a similar calorie count and saturated fat content as animal-based options. The bottom line: Just like you wouldn't eat a meat burger every day, plant-based alternatives are best enjoyed occasionally and in conjunction with an overall nutritious diet.

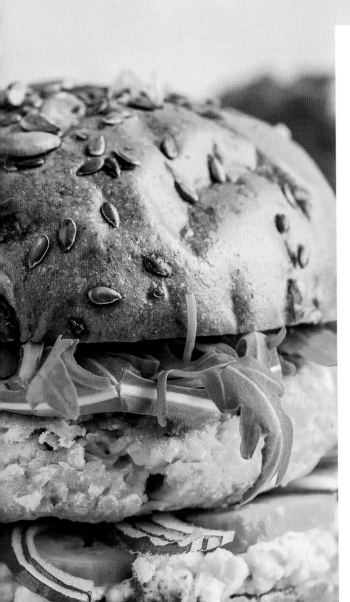

HOW TO PICK THE BEST MEAT SUBSTITUTES

THEY MAY SOUND HEALTHIER BUT BEWARE WHAT MAY BE HIDING INSIDE.

Chili-spiced walnut taco "meat," jackfruit pulled "pork" or portobello mushroom "burgers," anyone? Certain whole foods offer nearly identical flavor and texture substitutes for real meat—but most meat substitutes are highly processed. "That means they should not be mistaken as 'healthier,' but instead thought of as an alternative for those who are choosing to forgo meat," says Michelle Hyman, RD, a registered dietitian at Simple Solutions Weight Loss. "Most are made from soy, pea protein or wheat gluten, and as with anything, some are higher in fat, sodium and additives than others."

If you do opt for mock meat, keep an eye on the label, seeking out lower sodium and fewer ingredients. And keep in mind that most of the plant-based burgers with flavor and texture reminiscent of real meat are about on par, nutritionally, with 80/20 ground beef.

If you're more on the flexitarian side of plant-based eating, you can also find a wide variety of part-beef, part-vegetable blends in the burger case alongside those popular meat-like patties.

Look for whole plant ingredients on food labels.

As plant-based meats become more readily available, customers' attitudes and expectations are shifting, says Danny O'Malley, founder of Before the Butcher, which makes 100 percent plant-based burgers, pulled pork and more. "Even just a couple of years ago, our time was spent trying to educate the public. Today, they actively seek these products." Another major change: Companies are no longer marketing their products exclusively to vegans and vegetarians. Instead, the new wave of animal-product alternatives is intended to appeal to meat-eaters as well.

Quality Control

Availability isn't the only thing that's improved in the past few years—taste and consistency have, too. Long gone are the days when people had to suffer through underwhelming veggie burgers with a mouthfeel and flavor more akin to chomping down on cardboard than an Angus burger. The new generation of meat alternatives smell, sizzle and even "bleed" (thanks to beet juice extract) like the real deal. And the juicy, chewy, downright meaty consistency can fool even die-hard carnivores.

The convincing taste and texture is thanks to ingredients such as textured wheat protein, pea-based protein and soy protein, which form the base of many meat-alternative products. Food scientists then add in seasonings and other ingredients to perfect not only the taste, but also the appearance—for example, plant-based fats that mimic marbling in a burger or crisp up in a fake bacon.

"The bite, chew, taste, look and smell have evolved in such a way that it is difficult to tell them from animal-based products when they are included in a recipe or built like a burger would be, on a bun," says

O'Malley, referring to customers' reactions to his meatless products.

Taste is indeed top of mind for consumers. In 2016, Impossible Foods—maker of the Impossible Burger—asked people why they would purchase plant-based meat. The top response: The product has to taste good. And when the survey was repeated three years later, taste was still first on the list.

The Sustainability Factor

Interestingly, when Impossible Foods conducted that 2019 survey, customers' third reason for purchasing plant-based foods was one that hadn't even made the top 10 in 2016: a concern for sustainability. "The biggest change in consumer reception is awareness that 'meat is heat,' and that eating plants carries a vastly lower CO_2 footprint than eating animals," says a representative for Impossible Foods.

Even seafood lovers who are concerned about sustainability and the overfishing of our oceans now have alternate options. Companies like Good Catch Foods and Ocean Hugger Foods are bringing plant-based tuna (legume-based water-packed "tuna" and tomato-based "raw tuna," respectively), to people's plates, along with "crab" cakes and other fishy fare.

The Future of Meat Alternatives

While not plant-based, an intriguing trend to keep an eye on is lab-grown meat, which uses animal-derived muscle tissue, blurring the lines of what's considered vegetarian.

Innovation will inevitably continue to explode in the plant-based market as companies aim to make meat alternatives that are gamier and generally more delicious. More variety, amped-up flavor, and less harm to animals and the environment—seems like a win for all.

Milking It

Similar to the meat-alternatives market, the dairy-alternatives market is also quickly growing, and is expected to reach almost $41 billion by 2025, according to a report from Grand View Research, Inc. Whether you choose soy, oat, almond, coconut or another type of milk alternative, these plant-based beverages can be part of a healthy diet, says Michael Smith, MD. "Dairy-milk alternatives are fortified to provide the nutrients that traditionally come from dairy, namely calcium and vitamin D." Here, four things to know about nondairy milk.

YOU SHOULD READ THE LABEL

Some milk alternatives pack in sugar. "Make sure to choose unsweetened varieties to avoid the added sugars in the sweetened versions," says Smith.

OAT AND SOY MAY BE THE MOST SUSTAINABLE

Research from the University of Oxford found that producing oat and soy milks uses less land and less water than other milk alternatives, like rice and almond. But all nondairy milks have less of an environmental impact than dairy milk.

YOU CAN COOK WITH THEM

Most unsweetened, unflavored nondairy milks can be swapped cup for cup when cooking and baking. If your recipe calls for whole milk, higher-fat milk alternatives (like cashew or coconut) might be best.

KIDS SHOULD AVOID THEM

New guidelines say that plant-based milks shouldn't replace dairy milks for kids under 5, due to the nutrients their bodies need at that age.

NO COWS WERE INVOLVED IN THE MAKING OF THESE CREAMY MILKS.

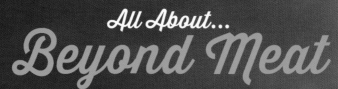

All About...
Beyond Meat

**THE COMPANY BEHIND THE FAMOUS BEYOND BURGER
IS CHANGING THE WAY AMERICA GRILLS, ONE BURGER (OR SAUSAGE) AT A TIME.**

HOW THE COMPANY STARTED
As a child, CEO Ethan Brown spent his summers on a family farm. The experience caused him to reconsider eating meat. In 2009, Beyond Meat was born. The company has received venture funding from Bill Gates, the Humane Society and others, and in 2013, PETA named Beyond Meat its company of the year.

WHAT'S ON THE MENU
Plant-based burgers, beef, sausage, crumbles and more

LET'S TALK ABOUT THAT BURGER...
The fan-favorite Beyond Burger gets its realistic, meaty texture from a process that heats, cools and adds pressure to plant-based proteins (the protein comes from peas, mung beans and rice). Coconut oil and potato starch are added to provide juiciness and a chewy bite, while cocoa butter provides a meat-like marbled appearance. Fruit- and vegetable-based colors and natural flavors are also added to give the Beyond Meat burger an authentic look and taste.

NUTRITION KNOW-HOW
With 20 grams of protein per patty (and 290 calories), the Beyond Burger has more protein than a 4-ounce, 80 percent lean/20 percent fat beef burger. It also delivers more iron and less saturated fat and total fat than the beef burger.

ECO EFFECT
Compared to producing a 4-ounce beef burger, the Beyond Burger uses 99 percent less land and about 50 percent less energy. It also generates 90 percent fewer greenhouse gas emissions.

AVAILABILITY
Beyond Meat is now available in 50-plus countries in more than 58,000 outlets, including Whole Foods, Publix, Kroger, Walmart and other supermarkets.

All About...
Impossible Foods

THE IMPOSSIBLE BURGER IS SHOWING UP NOT ONLY ON FAMILY DINNER TABLES, BUT ALSO ON RESTAURANT MENUS ACROSS THE COUNTRY.

HOW THE COMPANY STARTED
CEO Patrick Brown came up with the idea to create Impossible Foods when he was on sabbatical from his position as a biochemistry professor at Stanford University School of Medicine. He realized he could use his training and knowledge to make plant-based meat alternatives that would be better for both consumers and the environment. In 2011, he founded Impossible Foods.

WHAT'S ON THE MENU
Burgers, pork and sausage

LET'S TALK ABOUT THAT BURGER...
Impossible Burgers start with heme, an essential molecule found in both plants and animals (it's what gives meat that, well, meaty taste). Impossible Foods takes heme from the root of soybean plants, inserts it into genetically engineered yeast, and then ferments it to create the heme that's used to flavor the burgers. Soy and potato proteins add a meaty bite, and coconut and sunflower oils allow the burger to sizzle on the grill.

NUTRITION KNOW-HOW
One burger clocks in at 240 calories, with 14 grams of total fat and 19 grams of protein.

ECO EFFECT
Compared with making an animal-based burger, the Impossible Burger uses 96 percent less land and 87 percent less water, and generates 89 percent less greenhouse gas emissions. The company is working toward getting U.S. Green Business Council Zero Waste Certification.

AVAILABILITY
In addition to being served up in multiple restaurants, the Impossible Burger can be purchased at Walmart, Trader Joe's, Wegmans (select markets), Safeway (select markets) and Gelson's Markets in California.

Whether you have a meat-and-potatoes partner or kiddos who can't stand green stuff, getting your family on board with a plant-based diet can be tricky. Here's how to get your whole crew eating more plants—and loving it!

Cooking for a

PLAN A PLANT-BASED MEAL IN ADVANCE AND GIVE EVERYONE A TASK THEY CAN DO TO HELP GET DINNER ON THE TABLE.

Crowd

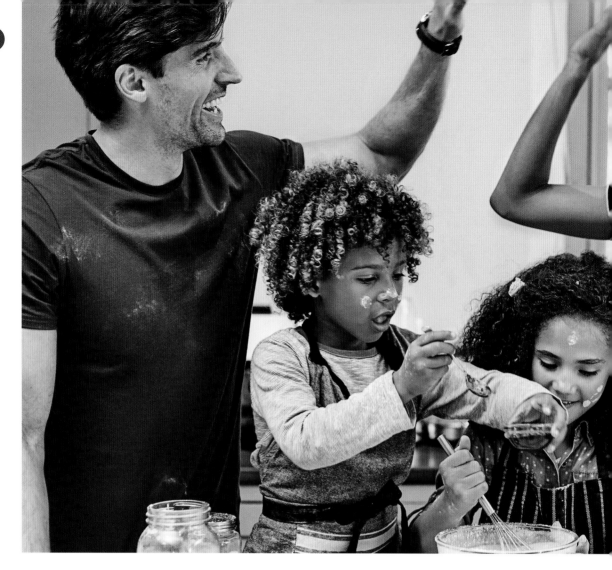

If your decision to go plant-based was met with a loud "yuck!" from the rest of your family, don't despair. There's no need to start cooking separate meals to please your partner's and kids' palates (hey, you've got enough on your to-do list!). After all, you likely want your loved ones to benefit from the same health boosts that come with increasing the consumption of plant-based foods. And you're not alone: One survey found that 75 percent of moms regularly use plant-based alternatives, and 66 percent say that they do so for health and nutrition reasons.

So what's a parent to do if tofu and almond milk are getting a big thumbs-down? First, don't panic. Experts say that with some smart (and yes, a few sneaky) tips, you can get your crew to gobble down plant-based meals.

When in Doubt, Add Seasoning

"It's all about flavor and spices," says Shiara van Ast Gore, head chef of BBVeganLtd, a café in Chichester, England, and head chef for KC Ubuntu Retreats, a series of health and wellness events based out of California. "If you treat vegetables as the

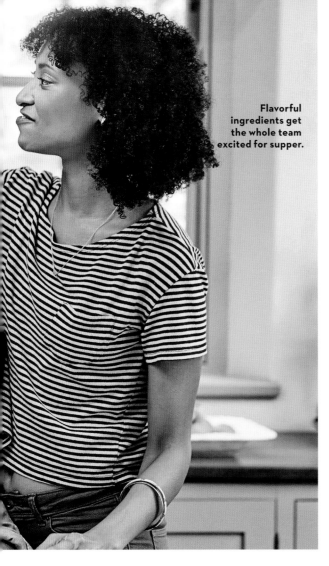

Flavorful ingredients get the whole team excited for supper.

Get Crafty

Slowly add plant-based foods into meals to help your family's taste buds adjust. For example, add finely chopped mushrooms to a favorite burger recipe or toss spiralized zucchini, also known as zoodles, into spaghetti dishes.

Focus on Variety

"I try to offer at least two vegetables with each meal," says Jenn Sebestyen, author of *The Meatless Monday Family Cookbook* and recipe blogger at veggieinspired.com. "I encourage my kids to take both, but if they only take one, that's fine. Don't give them the option of choosing none. Say, 'Do you want broccoli or green beans, or both?'"

Don't Forget the Sides

Getting complaints that plant-based isn't filling? Sebestyen says to start with a hearty dish (like bean chili or a pasta bake) and serve it with sides of salad and garlic bread or cornbread. "It rounds out the meal and everyone walks away full and happy."

Get the Kids Involved

Research shows that children who help out with meal prep are more likely to like fruits and veggies than kids who don't lend a hand with the cooking. Sebestyen suggests giving kids age-appropriate tasks, like washing produce and peeling carrots.

Head to the Store Together

Just like it's a great idea to get your children cooking in the kitchen, you can also involve them in choosing which recipe to make for dinner, as well as food shopping. "Ask them to pick out one new vegetable to try each time," suggests Sebestyen. "Kids are more likely to try something new when it is their idea."

main event, and flavor and spice them as you would a piece of chicken, then you are off to a good start." Stock your kitchen with a do-it-all spice, like McCormick Perfect Pinch Vegetable Seasoning or Trader Joe's Everyday Seasoning.

Play With Your Food!

Use cookie cutters to transform slices of firm tofu into fun shapes. Then toss them in a mouthwatering marinade, roast in the oven or in an air fryer, and serve with a dipping sauce, suggests van Ast Gore. It's a surefire way to get kids excited.

3 SMART SWAPS FOR EASY MEALS

GET EVERYONE TO EAT MORE VEGGIES WITH THESE HACKS.

**INSTEAD OF A BURGER
TRY A PORTOBELLO MUSHROOM
HOW TO MAKE IT** To give the mushrooms a meatier texture, remove the stems and bake the caps at 350°F for 10 to 15 minutes until they expel some of their moisture, then fry or cook them as you wish, says chef Shiara van Ast Gore.

Portobellos have a meat-like flavor—and they fit perfectly on a bun!

INSTEAD OF SPAGHETTI
TRY ZOODLES
HOW TO MAKE IT Use a spiralizer, mandoline or julienne peeler to slice up zucchini, carrots or whatever vegetable or fruit you want to use. Salt the noodles and let them sit in a colander for about 10 minutes, then rinse, pat dry and sauté over medium heat for 3 minutes. Toss in sauce before serving, if desired.

Zoodles take on whatever flavors you pair them with.

Save prep time by purchasing premade cauliflower rice.

INSTEAD OF RICE
TRY CAULIFLOWER RICE
HOW TO MAKE IT Wash, dry and remove greens, then grate cauliflower into rice-sized pieces. Eat raw, or sauté in a skillet over medium heat for 5 minutes or until tender (cover the skillet with a lid). Season and enjoy!

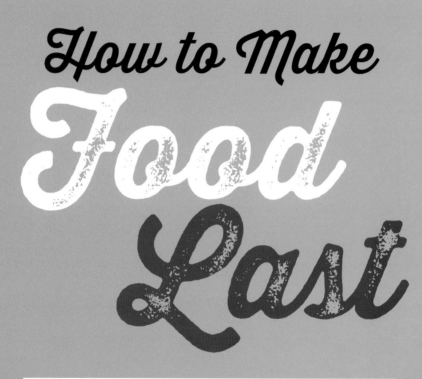

How to Make *Food* *Last*

Getting smart about your shopping list will not only stretch your budget, it will also help minimize waste.

A WHOLE-FOOD DIET IS SUPER HEALTHY— BUT WITHOUT PRESERVATIVES, FOOD SPOILS FASTER.

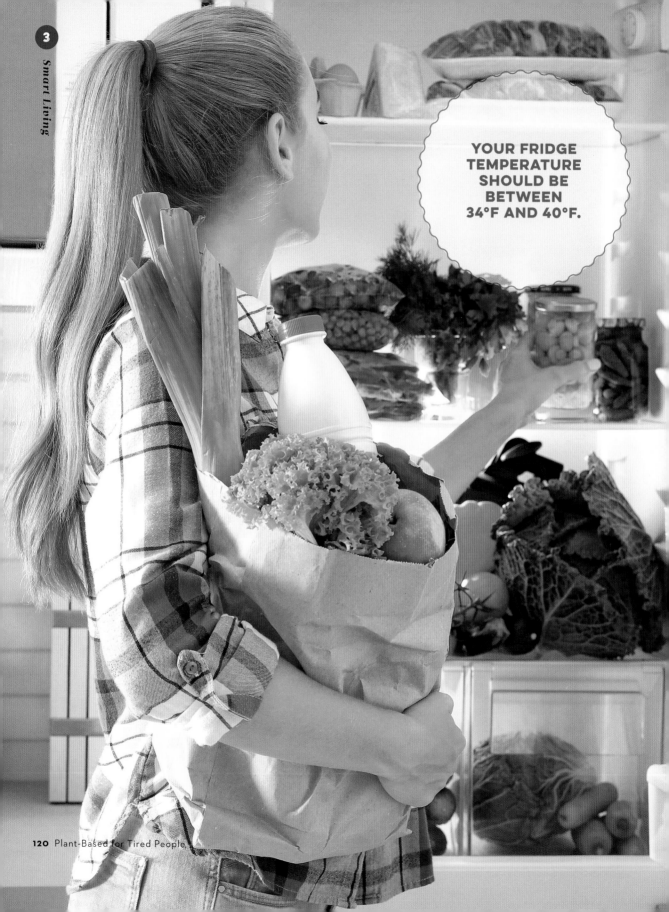

YOUR FRIDGE TEMPERATURE SHOULD BE BETWEEN 34°F AND 40°F.

The global pandemic and initial shutdown in 2020 was a wake-up call about how quickly food supplies can shift. With store shelves picked clean of staples and budgets suddenly pinched for many, it was more important than ever to make smart choices and to try to stretch the time between grocery trips. But establishing good buying habits will always serve you well, especially considering food waste in general is a huge issue: Each year, we waste nearly $162 billion in food, according to the USDA; that's a third of the food supply just tossed into the garbage, either at stores or in homes. In fact, the typical American family of four throws more than 1,000 pounds of food into the garbage every year (that's about 20 pounds a week!).

Food tastes better when it's fresh, but produce, bread and dairy spoil easily. To avoid living off canned beans and frozen peas, use these tips to enjoy everything the farmers market or grocery store has to offer, while still reducing waste and saving money.

1 Plan Ahead

Before you hit the store, figure out your meals for the week and determine what you need to purchase, then stick to your list, says Claudia Sidoti, head chef at HelloFresh. (A recent study published in *Resources, Conservation & Recycling* found that meal-kit delivery services like HelloFresh, which send preportioned ingredients, actually involve less food waste and environmental impact than store-bought meals—even when you factor in packaging.) If something comes up during the week and you end up eating out more than you anticipated, many perishables can last in the freezer, with little to no prep (keep containers on hand for storage).

2 Buy Right

While "ugly" produce is cheaper (there are produce-subscription boxes that specialize in reject, imperfect fruits and vegetables), if a piece of produce is bruised or damaged, it could spoil quicker. If you think you'll eat it fast, then don't be swayed by an unusual appearance; it will taste the same. (You can easily cut around bruises.)

3 Store It Properly

Tomatoes, potatoes and onions should never be stored in the fridge, but melons, apricots, strawberries, cruciferous veggies, leafy greens, zucchini and cherries should be refrigerated from the get-go. Peaches, kiwi and nectarines can stay out until they ripen.

In the fridge, utilize your crispers (see No. 4) and resist the urge to wash everything before you put it away. You should wash produce right before you use it, not before you store it (even organic produce), since that can speed spoilage. Store greens in a resealable plastic bag with a damp paper towel, being careful to remove as much air from the bag as possible, says Sidoti. "Date and label any cut veggies and remember to practice FIFO [first in, first out]." (Date your freezer foods too; they can be difficult to identify.)

To store produce in the freezer, there are two approaches. For veggies, blanch them for a couple of minutes, then immediately plunge them into an ice bath. Let dry, and then spread on a cookie sheet and place it in the freezer. Once frozen, place produce in a sealed container with as little air as possible.

Fruit doesn't need to be blanched; sliced fruit may last better if you top it with sugar first. Berries, however, can be frozen without sugar. Freeze the fruit on a

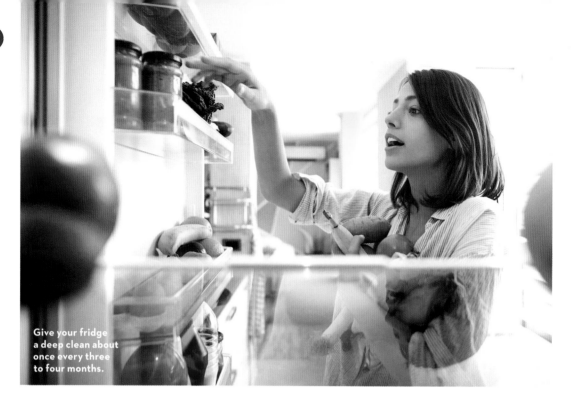

Give your fridge a deep clean about once every three to four months.

sheet pan, and then transfer to an airtight container—and date it—before storing.

4 Know Your Fridge

The coldest areas in the refrigerator are usually the lowermost shelves (this can change depending on your appliance, but in general, cold air sinks). The door is the warmest; don't store milk or eggs or anything that can spoil easily there. Also, one crisper drawer is for fruit and the other is for veggies, right? Wrong! One is typically for low-humidity produce and the other is for high-humidity items (a lever may let you adjust airflow in the bin).

Store apples, pears, avocados, melon and stone fruits in the low-humidity drawer (or adjust the setting to low); that will allow the fruit to "breathe" (they emit a natural gas called ethylene that can speed ripening of other produce). Make the other drawer high-humidity and store your greens in there, as well as unripe bananas, strawberries and cruciferous veggies (cabbage, broccoli, kale and cauliflower). Be sure not to overcrowd your drawers, says Sidoti. It can contribute to damage and reduce air circulation, which can speed spoilage. Plus, if you can't see it, you won't eat it.

5 Save With Bulk Purchases

Whether it's meat or produce, "buying in bulk can be great [if you'll use it]," says Sidoti. "Just portion it out and freeze what you can't use yet." She uses this approach with bread, too: "You can cut whole loaves into quarters and then wrap it well and freeze."

6 Get Creative

If produce is starting to spoil, cook it and then toss anything left into meals the rest of the week. Root-to-stem eating will allow you to use all parts of produce, too, like sautéing the leaves on kohlrabi or pickling watermelon rind.

Cycle your stash so the most recently purchased foods go toward the back.

"Can I Still Eat That?"

Use-by dates on foods are notoriously conservative, which can lead to unnecessary food waste. (The yogurt that says it expired last week? It's still good!) "Don't assume things are bad if they're past their use-by date," says HelloFresh chef Claudia Sidoti. "Depending on the item, it's likely still good. Look for signs of spoilage first: color, mold, odor and of course, off-putting taste." (FYI: These won't tip you off to bugs that can cause food poisoning.)

Use-by dates are more about food quality— when it will be at its best, flavor-wise—than safety. In addition, the sell-by dates are for the retailer. The use-by dates are for the consumer.

Not sure what you can get away with? The FoodKeeper app (free for both Android and iOS devices) will tell you when you should really throw out more than 400 food and beverage items, whether they're stored in the fridge or freezer.

SMART STORAGE TIPS

MAKE YOUR FRESH FARE LAST EVEN LONGER WITH THESE EASY FIXES.

If you're planning on serving certain veggies later in the week, buy them on the firm side.

FOOD	STORE IT THIS WAY	FOR THIS LONG
AVOCADO (ALREADY CUT OPEN)	Brush with lemon juice and seal in an airtight container to keep it from turning brown.	Several days with good storage
BREAD	Fresh: in a plastic bag or foil on the counter or in a bread box. Commercial bread: Keep in the fridge. In the freezer, use a resealable plastic bag.	Up to a few days on the counter (and then think: breadcrumbs, croutons and French toast!). In the fridge, a loaf may last two or three weeks.
CHEESE (HARD)	Wrap it in wax paper before putting it in plastic wrap and storing in the fridge.	Up to six months in the refrigerator, unopened. If opened, about a month
MILK	Keep it in the fridge or freezer.	In the fridge, it will last five to seven days past the sell-by date (give it the sniff test); in the freezer, six months
CELERY	Wrap it with foil and store it in the high-humidity crisper drawer, or cut the stalks into smaller chunks and store in water.	A few weeks
FRESH HERBS	Wrap with a damp towel in a sealed bag.	A week or more
TOMATOES	Store in a cool, dry place (not the fridge).	A week
RICE	Uncooked, in a tightly closed container	A year or longer
COFFEE	In an airtight container in the pantry	Three to five weeks after opening
OLIVE OIL	In a well-sealed bottle, in a dark cabinet	Up to six months
EGGS	Keep them in their original container in the coldest part of the refrigerator.	Three to five weeks (in shells)
FRESH PASTA	In a sealed container	Up to six months

TO AVOID
CONTAMINANTS,
MAKE SURE YOUR
SUPPLEMENT
IS NSF OR
USP CERTIFIED.

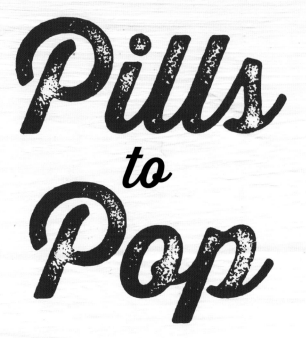

Pills to Pop

Diet is the best way to get your nutrients—but when that doesn't work, these supplements may help you sleep better, avoid getting sick and more.

Nutritionists recommend getting your daily doses of fiber, vitamins and minerals through diet because that's the way nature intended. Nutrients in food come wrapped up with other nutrients, which may improve their overall function and benefit. In plants, it's even more important, because vitamins and minerals are surrounded by phytonutrients—antioxidants, polyphenols and other health-promoting compounds. Although it seems like a no-brainer, when you extract the one crucial nutrient—like lycopene from tomatoes, or resveratrol from grapes—and put it in a pill, it often doesn't work the same way as it might in food. But sometimes you need an extra boost. The following can help plug some surprising nutrient holes.

Magnesium

TAKE IT IF you're constipated, having trouble sleeping or having muscle spasms.

This multitasking mineral is found in every cell and has a role in countless bodily functions, including energy metabolism and bone-building (a lack of it can contribute to osteoporosis). According to a 2018 study published in *Open Heart*, up to 30 percent of the population may be low in magnesium. The study authors speculated that a lack of minerals in soil used to grow food and a diet high in refined foods can exacerbate a magnesium deficiency.

FIND IT IN almonds, spinach, peanuts, cashews and black beans

DAILY DOSE up to 420 mg

Vitamin B12

TAKE IT IF you're on antacids or proton pump inhibitors (PPIs).

The B vitamins in general are involved with energy metabolism (among several other functions) and they tend to hang out together. Vitamin B12, aka cyanocobalamin in supplement form, plays a key role in nerve function, blood-cell health and the creation of genetic material. It also helps break down levels of homocysteine, a compound that can contribute to inflammation, especially in the arteries.

According to the Harvard T.H. Chan School of Public Health, up to 15 percent of the population may have a vitamin B12 deficiency, and it's more common as you get older. The vitamin gets liberated from food in the stomach, with the help of hydrochloric acid. As you age, you make less stomach acid. That's also why people who are chronic users of antacids and other drugs that decrease stomach acid are at risk for a deficiency. Finally, since B12 is found naturally only in animal products (it's added to other foods), vegetarians and vegans can run low on the crucial vitamin.

FIND IT IN clams, liver, trout, canned tuna, salmon and nutritional yeast

DAILY DOSE 2.4 mcg (supplements contain way more, but you'll only absorb a fraction)

Vitamin C

TAKE IT IF you're training for a race or feeling stressed.

This hardworking antioxidant vitamin has a sunny reputation, thanks in part to the citrus fruits it's found in. Many people keep it on hand to take at the first sign of a cold, for good reason. "I like to call it an immune surveillance optimizer," says physician and researcher Mark Moyad, MD, author of *The Supplement Handbook* and director of preventive/complementary and alternative medicine at the University of Michigan Medical Center. "It helps your immune system work smarter, not harder, and no supplement is cheaper or more effective at it."

Squeeze some vitamin C into your diet with a variety of citrusy fare.

Large studies have shown that it can help reduce the duration of the common cold by about 20 percent, and it can cut your risk of getting a cold in half when your system is being taxed or you're stressed, like when you're training for a marathon or buried in projects at work. Doctors have been giving this antioxidant vitamin to COVID-19 patients in high-dose IV drips, but the research is still out on whether it made a significant difference.

FIND IT IN red and green peppers, oranges, strawberries, broccoli and kiwi

DAILY DOSE The recommended daily intake is 75 mg (90 mg for men) but supplements always contain more than that. You can take 500 mg daily for no more than three months. If you're training for a marathon or some other tough event, take that dose twice daily for a few weeks beforehand. To minimize the risk of kidney stones, look for the calcium ascorbate form (Moyad prefers Ester-C).

Omega-3 Fatty Acids

TAKE THEM IF you have high triglycerides or don't eat fish.

Also known as PUFAs (polyunsaturated fatty acids), omega-3s have anti-inflammatory benefits and help with cell structure, immune function, hormone production and energy metabolism. There are three main types of omega-3s: ALA (alpha-linolenic acid), DHA (docosahexaenoic acid) and EPA (eicosapentaenoic acid). The latter two are found in fish and seafood; ALA is found in plants. It's converted into EPA and DHA so it's easier to get your omega-3s in DHA and EPA. The supplement form (aka fish oil) has had inconsistent research supporting it. It can help reduce triglyceride levels (not LDLs) and in 2018 the results of the VITAL trial, which looked at vitamin D3 and

omega-3 supplementation for cancer and cardiovascular disease, found that people who supplemented with omega-3s saw a 28 percent reduced risk of heart attack. (The people who benefited most were African Americans, who saw a 77 percent reduced risk of heart attack, and people who ate less than 1.5 servings of fish a week.) It did not have an impact on cancer prevention. Supplementation may also have a beneficial impact on cognitive function.

FIND THEM IN cold-water fish (salmon, mackerel, tuna, herring, sardines) as well as flaxseeds, chia seeds, plant oils and walnuts

DAILY DOSE If you can't add fish to your diet twice a week, aim for 1,000 mg to 4,000 mg per day of EPA and DHA.

Probiotics

TAKE THEM IF you're prone to upper respiratory tract infections or will be traveling to an area with poor sanitation or water quality.

The colonies of beneficial bacteria in the GI tract seemingly have an impact on everything in the body, including digestion, mental health, immunity, weight loss, fertility and more. A healthy population of good bugs also helps keep bad bugs under control.

There are tons of studies underway looking at which strains do what in the body—and how—and whether taking them in pill form can make a difference in the gut. That's the big question. The American Gastroenterological Association recently issued its first-ever guidelines for probiotic use in GI disorders and found that, based on extensive studies, there's not enough evidence to recommend using probiotics to treat conditions like IBS, ulcerative colitis or Crohn's disease. (If you're taking them and seeing a benefit, however, there's no reason to stop.)

L. RHAMNOSUS GG, S. BOULARDII AND B. BIFIDUM ARE SOME OF THE MOST COMMON (AND MOST STUDIED) PROBIOTICS.

One review and analysis of research found them to be helpful in reducing the risk of getting an upper respiratory tract infection; they shortened the duration of the infection and antibiotic use. For frequent overseas travelers, a product like Culturelle can reduce the risk of traveler's diarrhea by a whopping 85 percent, according to studies. "I still say that if you get enough fiber and potassium you'll be able to make plenty of probiotics without having to take a pill," says Moyad. (If you're under a doctor's care for a health condition, check to make sure a probiotic is safe.)

FIND THEM IN kefir and yogurt

DAILY DOSE Follow the package instructions. If you're going to a place with sketchy sanitation, start two to five days before your trip. Whatever you take, switch it up every couple of months so you don't encourage an overgrowth of one type of bacteria.

Calcium Carbonate

TAKE IT IF you have PMS.

There's less need to supplement this mineral these days, thanks to all the fortified foods that are available, says Moyad. Plus, there is some contradictory research about calcium supplementation: Some studies show benefits, while others conclude there may be some harm. Where it does show good benefit is for PMS. The large Premenstrual Syndrome Study Group trial found that after three months, almost 50 percent of women taking calcium carbonate reported reduced PMS symptoms (pain, depression, fatigue and edema) compared to those downing a placebo.

FIND IT IN dark leafy greens, soy products (tofu, edamame), fortified cereals and dairy

DAILY DOSE 1,200 mg in divided doses. (Check with your doctor first if you're on any medications or have heart disease.)

Taking a multi can help you make sure you're not deficient in any one area.

Cover Your Bases

Check your cupboards, and odds are you have a multivitamin in there. (Whether you take it regularly is another question!) There's been so much conflicting research on multis, it's hard to know whether they're worth the money.

Research does support at least one brand: Centrum Silver has been shown to help reduce the risk of cancer (for men) and cataracts (the leading cause of blindness in the world), says Mark Moyad, MD, author of *The Supplement Handbook*. Because dosages of the vitamins and minerals it contains have changed over the years since the study, he says a children's multi should be very similar in content.

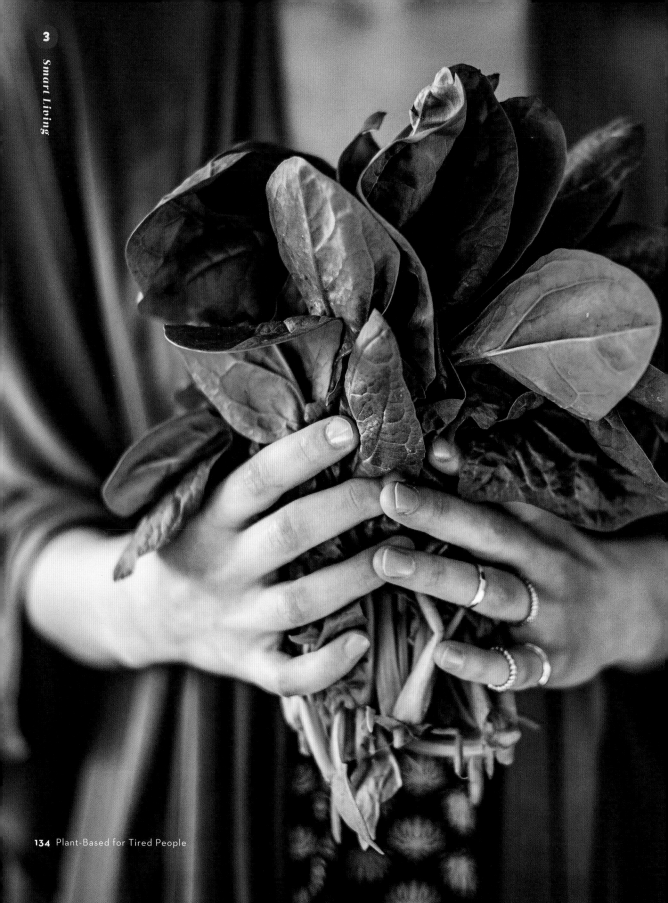

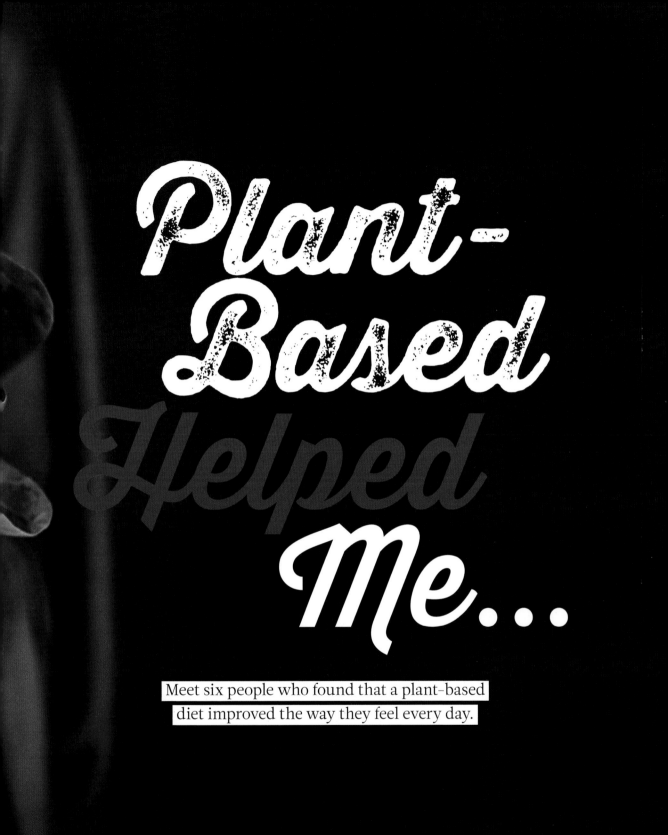

Plant-Based Helped Me...

Meet six people who found that a plant-based diet improved the way they feel every day.

Athletes should
focus on plant
foods that are
nutrient dense.

...Improve My Running

CHRISTIAN TANNER; AUSTIN, TX

"After just one full day on a plant-based diet, I noticed that the swelling I usually experience in my legs after running completely went away. I also found that my energy became more consistent through the day. The biggest benefit I've noticed is how I've put on more muscle than ever before. I'm so grateful that I made the decision to switch to a plant-based diet."

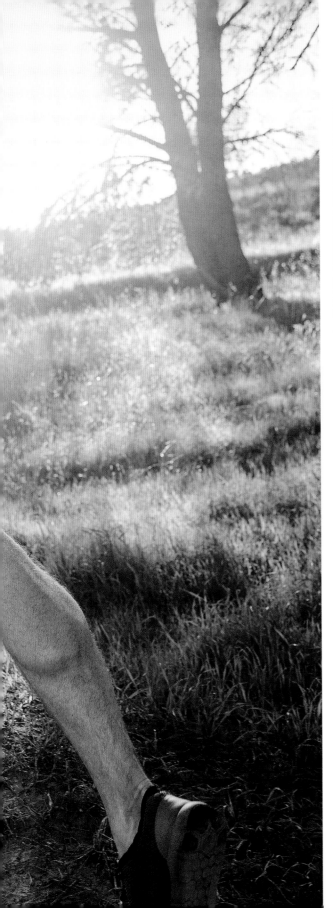

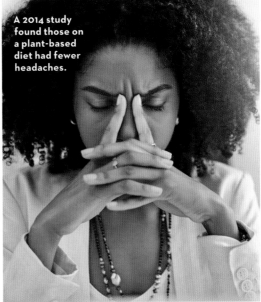

A 2014 study found those on a plant-based diet had fewer headaches.

...Ease My Migraines

JENAY ROSE; LOS ANGELES

"Becoming incredibly passionate about yoga led me to adopt a more conscious lifestyle, which naturally brought me to a plant-based diet. I immediately no longer felt sick after I ate. But there were unexpected impacts, too: My anxiety eased up and my migraines became much less frequent and severe. I'm so glad to have finally found some relief!"

...Overcome My Endometriosis Pain

ELIZABETH COE; DELRAY BEACH, FL

"I have endometriosis, and since changing my diet five years ago, I have experienced significantly fewer instances of pain, which I believe is directly linked to eating more anti-inflammatory plant-based foods. For example, I used to experience endometriosis pain once a month. Now I have it only a few times a year—and it's not nearly as painful as it once was."

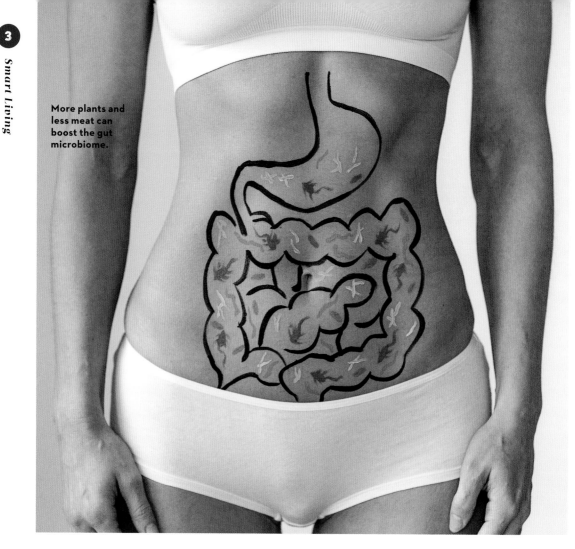

More plants and less meat can boost the gut microbiome.

...Improve My Digestion

ASHLEY KITCHENS SWANSON; DURHAM, NC

"I've had chronic constipation since I was little. As a child, I remember getting suppositories and using a lot of over-the-counter laxatives and fiber products. A few years ago, I started connecting the dots. When I ate dairy products, I felt miserable afterward, so I tried going plant-based. I reached for hummus instead of cheese and snacked on fresh fruit rather than yogurt. It worked! My constipation and the accompanying discomfort eased up. I grew up having a glass of milk with every meal, but consuming more water and plant milk is easier on my digestive system. I'm so much happier now!"

...Get Better Skin

LESLIE NIFOUSSI; JUPITER, FL

"I started my plant-based journey 15 years ago, long before things like 'tofurkey' were mainstream. I wasn't unhealthy, nor was I looking to lose weight, but I was in search of mental clarity and increased energy. One of the biggest positive impacts I've noticed has been the youthful and supple appearance of my skin; you can even say it glows! Thanks to cutting animal products out of my diet and eating more water-packed fruits and vegetables, as well as an increased amount of nuts, seeds and olive oil, my skin is now clear and smooth. I've even stopped wearing foundation!"

...Recover From Knee Surgery

MORGAN BALAVAGE; SANTA BARBARA, CA

"After I tore my ACL, a friend recommended that I try eating fewer animal products to help reduce the insane inflammation that plagued me for weeks before my surgery. I tried it for a few weeks and noticed a massive shift in my entire body. I felt lighter overall, and the swelling was definitely reduced. In the two-and-a-half years since I made the commitment to eating plant-based, I've lost 20 pounds, sleep better, smell better (really!), and overall have more energy throughout the day than I did when I was eating dairy and meat."

Less inflammation in the body can translate to less joint pain.

IN GOOD COMPANY

YOU'RE NOT THE ONLY ONE THINKING OF GOING PLANT-BASED! THESE CELEBS ALSO DECIDED TO ADOPT A VERSION OF THE DIET.

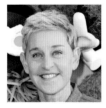
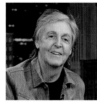
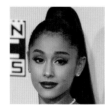
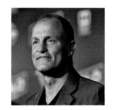
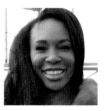

ELLEN DeGENERES
The talk-show host went vegan in 2008, and in 2019, she and her wife, Portia de Rossi, invested in the vegan brand Miyoko's Creamery.

PAUL McCARTNEY
The Beatles star is a vegan, and in 2017, he and his family launched *One Day a Week*, a short film that encourages people to give up animal products one day each week.

ARIANA GRANDE
The "thank u, next" singer has been on a macrobiotic vegan diet since 2013. She has said it makes her an all-around happier person.

WOODY HARRELSON
The actor has been vegan since he was 24 years old and has said one reason for the lifestyle change was that he would feel "knocked out" after eating burgers and steak.

VENUS WILLIAMS
The tennis pro adopted a plant-based diet after an autoimmune disease halted her career. She credits her new way of eating as something that helped her get back in the game.

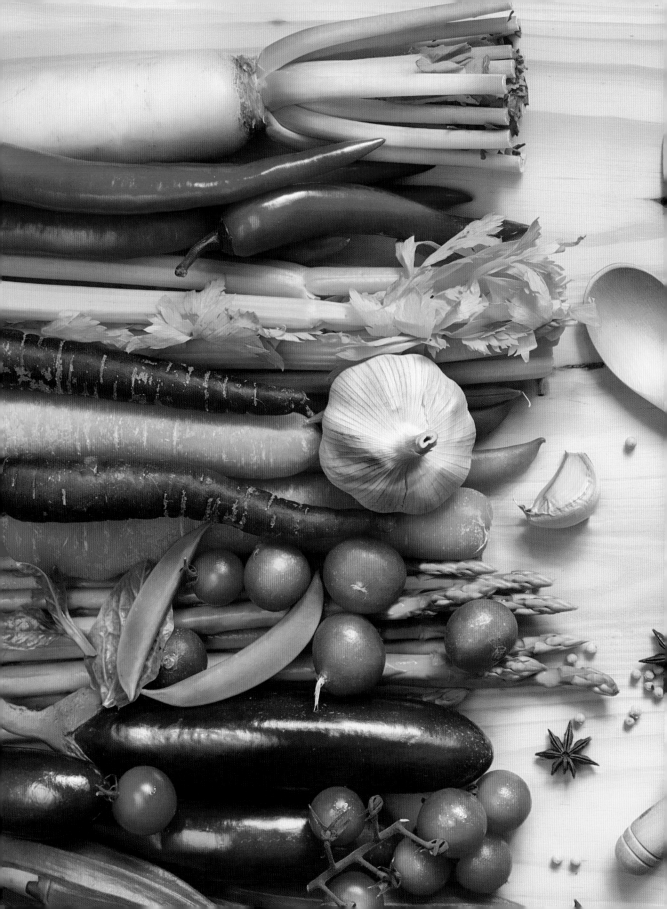

ENERGIZING RECIPES

Think you need meat to make a meal? No way!
As these 32 recipes show, there's
no shortage of flavor and taste on a plant-based diet.

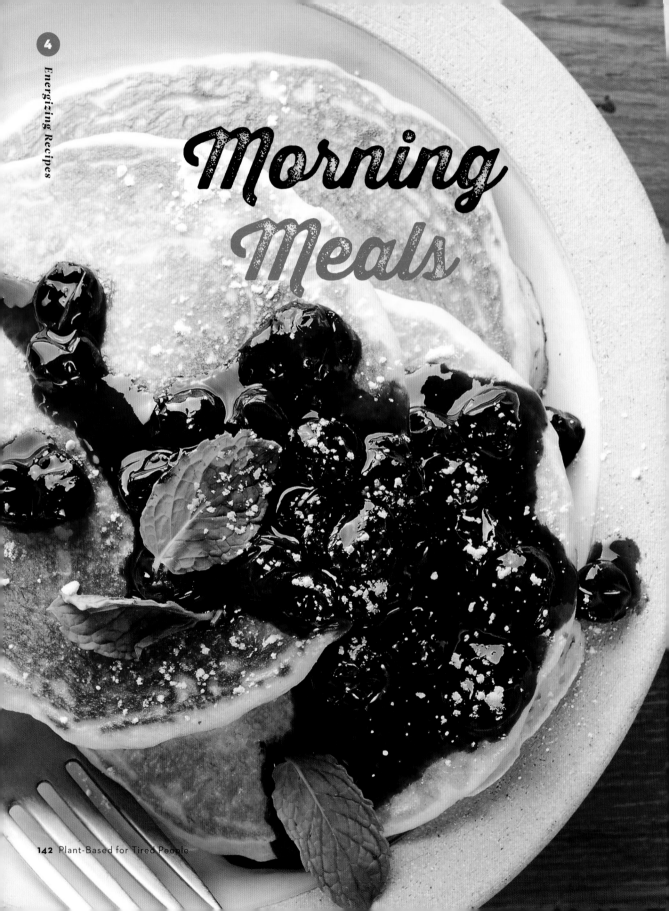

Morning Meals

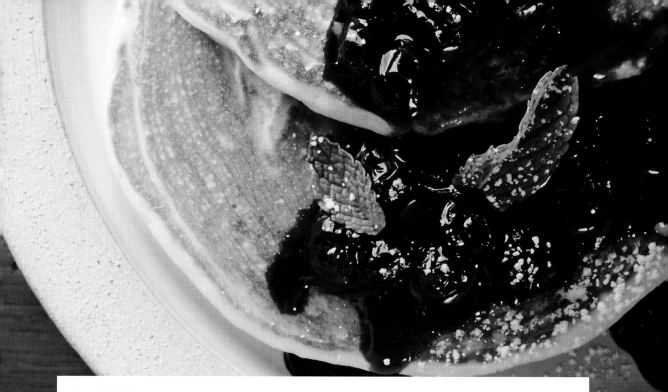

BUTTERMILK PANCAKES WITH BLUEBERRY SAUCE

These pancakes have a slightly crispy golden crust with a light, tender interior. Buttermilk has a delicious flavor and reacts with the baking soda for fluffier cakes. And the easy-to-make blueberry sauce is packed with antioxidants.

PREP 15 minutes
TOTAL 25 minutes
SERVINGS 2

INGREDIENTS

BLUEBERRY SAUCE

 1 cup fresh or frozen blueberries, divided
 1/3 cup water
 2 tablespoons sugar
 1/4 teaspoon vanilla extract
 1 1/2 teaspoons cornstarch dissolved in 1 tablespoon water

BLUEBERRY PANCAKES

 1 egg, beaten
 1 1/4 cups buttermilk
 1 1/4 cups all-purpose flour
 1 tablespoon sugar
 1 teaspoon baking powder
 1/2 teaspoon baking soda
 1/2 teaspoon kosher salt

INSTRUCTIONS

1 For sauce, in a small saucepan combine 3/4 cup blueberries, water, sugar and vanilla extract. Bring to a gentle boil over medium-high heat. Gently boil just until blueberries are soft and begin to fall apart.

2 Stir in the dissolved cornstarch-water mixture. Bring to boil; reduce heat to low. Gently simmer 2 to 3 minutes or until slightly thickened, stirring occasionally. (If sauce becomes too thick, continue cooking and stir in additional water, 1 tablespoon at a time, until desired consistency.) Remove saucepan from heat. Gently stir in remaining blueberries. Set sauce aside.

3 For pancakes, in a small bowl combine egg and buttermilk. In a medium bowl, combine remaining ingredients. Add buttermilk mixture to flour mixture. Stir just until moistened (batter will be lumpy).

4 Heat a lightly greased griddle or heavy skillet over medium-high heat. When griddle is hot, use a 1/4-cup measure to pour batter into griddle; spread batter if necessary. Cook over medium heat for 2 to 4 minutes, turning pancakes over when surface tops are bubbly and edges are slightly dry. Serve hot with warm blueberry sauce.

SAVORY YOGURT BOWL WITH RAW VEGETABLES

Greek yogurt is full of probiotics—the good bacteria that aids in restoring a healthy gut balance.

PREP 10 minutes
TOTAL 10 minutes
SERVINGS 1

INGREDIENTS

- 1   cup Greek yogurt
- 1   green onion, sliced
- 1   small carrot, cut into ribbons
- 1   small Persian cucumber, sliced in half-moons
- 1   large radish, sliced
- 6   cherry tomatoes, halved
- 1/4 cup micro parsley greens
- 1   teaspoon black chia seeds

INSTRUCTIONS

1 Place yogurt in a serving bowl.
2 Top with green onion, carrot, cucumber, radish and tomatoes.
3 Sprinkle with micro parsley greens and black chia seeds.

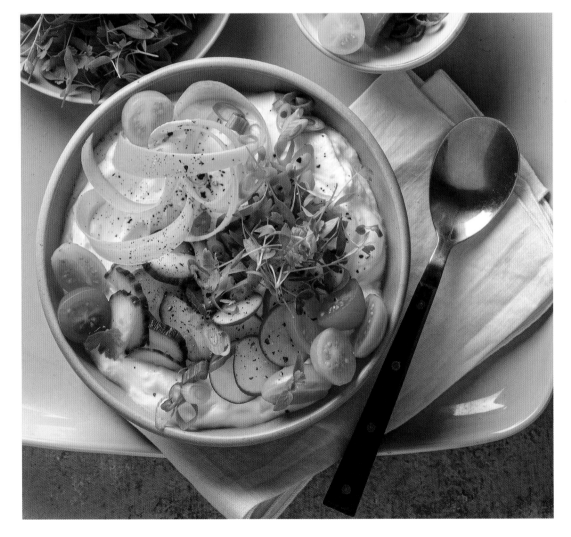

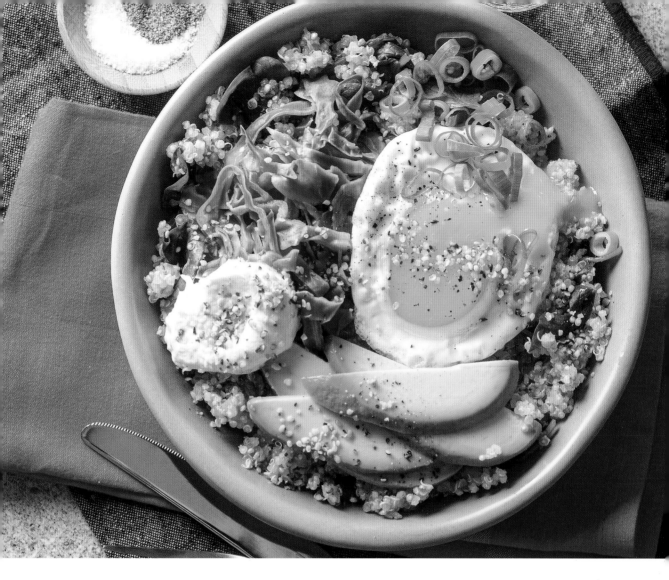

PROBIOTIC BREAKFAST BOWL

Quinoa works in many forms, but it's especially delicious as the base in a hearty and savory bowl like this one, which is packed with protein, probiotics and healthy fats.

PREP 10 minutes
TOTAL 30 minutes
SERVINGS 4

INGREDIENTS

- 1 cup uncooked quinoa
- 2 cups vegetable broth
- ½ teaspoon sea salt
- 2 cups baby spinach leaves
- 4 fried eggs
- 2 avocados, pitted and sliced
- 3 green onions, sliced
- 1 cup fermented purple cabbage or kimchi
- ¼ cup plain Greek yogurt
- 4 teaspoons hemp seeds

INSTRUCTIONS

1 In a medium saucepan, combine quinoa, vegetable broth and salt. Bring to a boil.
2 Cover; reduce heat and simmer 15 minutes or until liquid is absorbed.
3 Remove from heat and stir in spinach; cover and let stand 5 minutes.
4 Fluff with a fork and divide evenly among 4 bowls.
5 Top each bowl with a fried egg and equal amounts of avocado slices, green onion slices, fermented cabbage or kimchi, yogurt and hemp seeds.

OVERNIGHT OATS WITH BLUEBERRIES AND WALNUTS

Creamy and tart like yogurt, but higher in protein and probiotics, kefir is available in both dairy and nondairy versions.

PREP 5 minutes
TOTAL 5 minutes + 12 hours inactive
SERVINGS 1

INGREDIENTS

- 1 cup kefir
- 1/4 cup gluten-free oats, toasted
- 2 tablespoons black chia seeds
- 1/2 teaspoon vanilla extract
- 1 tablespoon blueberries
  Toppings: chopped walnuts, sunflower seeds

INSTRUCTIONS

1 In a pint-size mason jar with a lid, stir together kefir, toasted oats, black chia seeds and vanilla extract. Add remaining blueberries.

2 Refrigerate overnight.

3 Top with chopped walnuts and sunflower seeds.

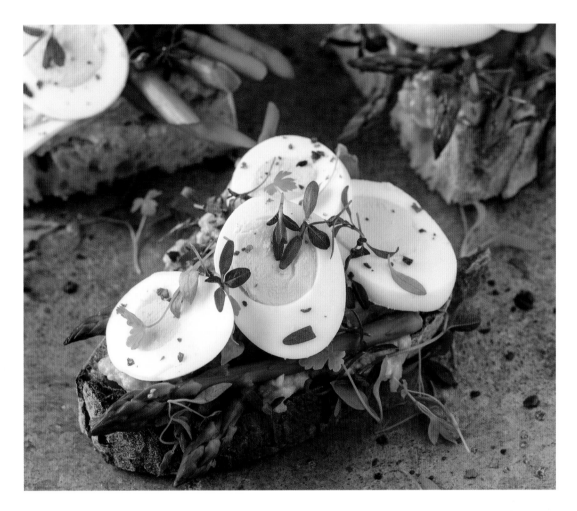

ASPARAGUS AND AVOCADO TOAST WITH HARD-BOILED EGGS

Asparagus is a rich source of folate and vitamins A, C and K, and pairs well with the avocado and eggs.

PREP 5 minutes
TOTAL 15 minutes
SERVINGS 4

INGREDIENTS

2   avocados
½   teaspoon sea salt
1   teaspoon lime juice
4   slices crusty sourdough bread, toasted
20 thin asparagus spears, trimmed and steamed
4   hard–boiled eggs, sliced
2   teaspoons Aleppo pepper
4   tablespoons microgreens or watercress

INSTRUCTIONS

1 Cut each avocado in half and remove pit. Scoop out the avocado flesh into a small bowl and mash with salt and lime juice.

2 Spread mixture evenly over the 4 toast pieces.

3 Top each toast with 5 asparagus spears and then with sliced eggs.

4 Sprinkle evenly with Aleppo pepper and microgreens or watercress to serve.

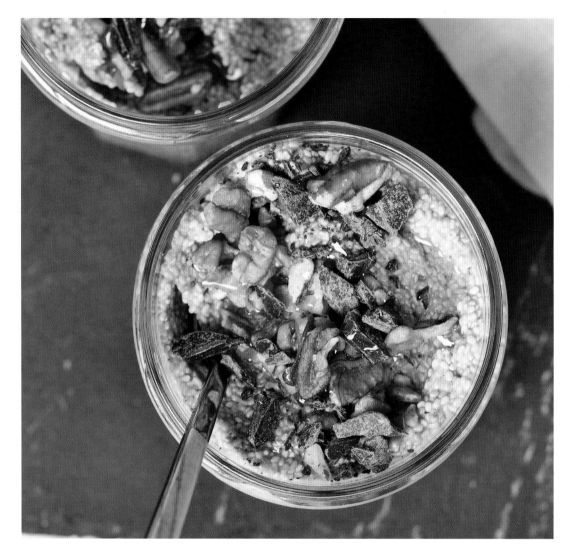

BREAKFAST CHIA-PUDDING BOWLS WITH CACAO NIBS AND PECANS

These bowls are full of fiber, good fats and protein. Make them the night before—that way, no matter how busy you are, there's no excuse for not having a healthy breakfast!

PREP 5 minutes
TOTAL 10 minutes + 12 hours inactive
SERVINGS 2

INGREDIENTS

- ¼ cup chia seeds
- 1 cup almond milk
- 2 teaspoons honey
- 1 tablespoon cacao nibs
- 1 tablespoon chopped pecans

INSTRUCTIONS

1 Divide chia seeds, almond milk and honey in 2 lidded jars. Cover and shake to mix.
2 Refrigerate overnight.
3 Top with cacao nibs and chopped pecans.

SHEET PAN ROASTED BABY BOK CHOY, TOMATOES AND EGGS

Bok choy is a good source of fiber, which feeds healthy gut bacteria. It also contains selenium, which is anti-inflammatory.

PREP 5 minutes
TOTAL 15 minutes
SERVINGS 3

INGREDIENTS

- 2 tablespoons olive oil
- 6 heads baby bok choy, halved
- 1 cup baby heirloom cherry tomatoes, halved
- 1/2 teaspoon salt
- 1/2 teaspoon black pepper
- 6 whole eggs

INSTRUCTIONS

1 Preheat oven to 375°F.
2 Brush sheet pan with olive oil.
3 Spread bok choy and tomatoes in pan; sprinkle with salt and pepper.
4 Make 6 wells in vegetable mixture and crack one egg in each well.
5 Bake for 6 minutes or until eggs are cooked to desired degree of doneness.

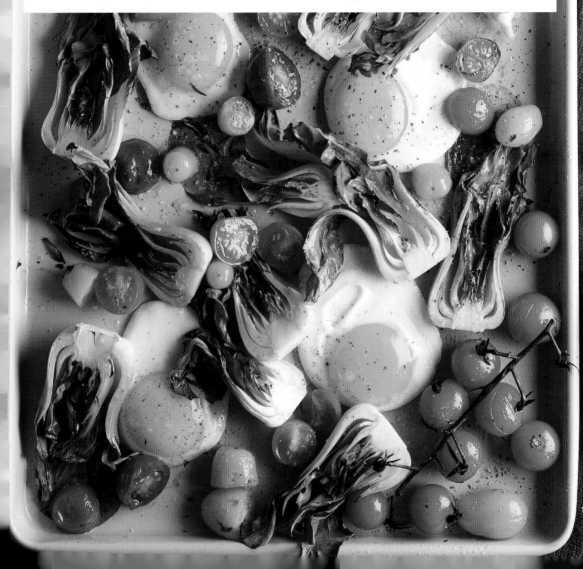

ALMOND PEANUT BUTTER BANANA TOAST

Add chia seeds to recipes when you can; they're nutrient dense and add a nutty taste.

PREP 5 minutes
TOTAL 5 minutes
SERVINGS 1

INGREDIENTS

- 1 tablespoon natural peanut butter
- 1 tablespoon almond butter
- $1/8$ teaspoon cinnamon
- 1 large slice gluten-free bread, toasted
- $1/2$ small banana, sliced
- $1/2$ teaspoon black chia seeds
  Toppings: chopped almonds, chopped peanuts

INSTRUCTIONS

1 In a small bowl, stir together peanut butter, almond butter and cinnamon until smooth.
2 Spread mixture on toasted bread.
3 Top with banana slices, chia seeds and nuts.

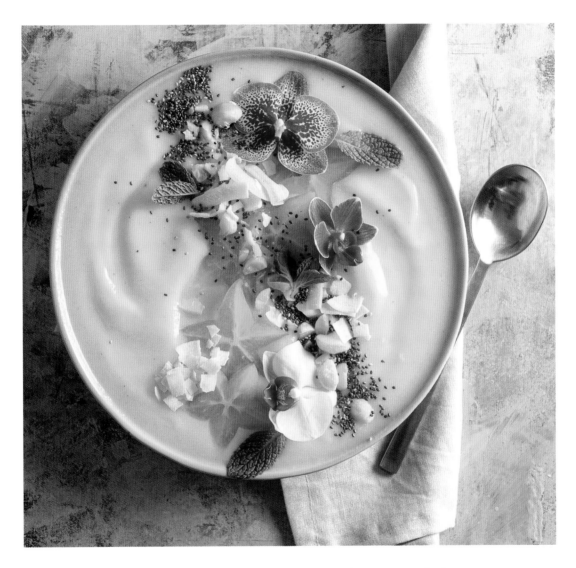

TROPICAL SMOOTHIE BOWL

Many smoothies start with frozen banana slices.
To ensure you always have some on hand, slice up a
bunch, put in zip-close bags and stash in the freezer.

PREP 5 minutes
TOTAL 5 minutes
SERVINGS 2

INGREDIENTS

- 2 bananas, sliced and frozen
- 2 cups frozen mango pieces
- 2 cups frozen pineapple pieces
- 2 cups coconut milk
  Toppings: star fruit, chopped macadamia nuts, toasted coconut flakes, black chia seeds, orchid blossoms

INSTRUCTIONS

1 In a blender, mix all ingredients except toppings until smooth.
2 Pour into bowls; garnish as desired.

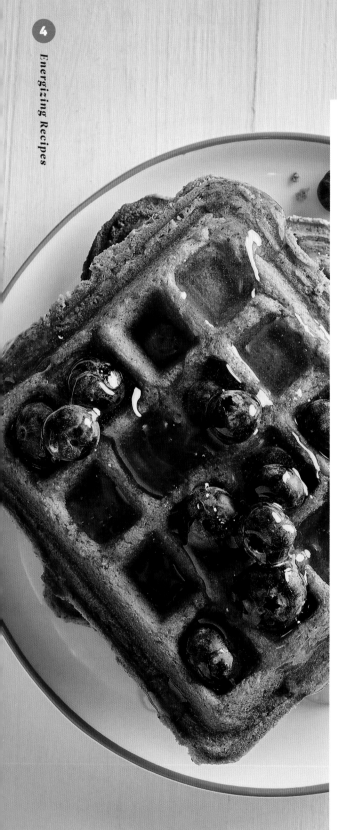

SPICED SWEET POTATO-BLUEBERRY WAFFLES

Blueberries and sweet potatoes are on the superfoods list—both are packed with antioxidants. Serve this topped with pure maple syrup, honey or agave syrup.

PREP 10 minutes
TOTAL 35 minutes
SERVINGS 2

INGREDIENTS

- 1   medium sweet potato, peeled and cubed
- 1   cup almond flour
- 2   tablespoons coconut flour
- 1   teaspoon ground cinnamon
- $^1/_2$ teaspoon ground nutmeg
- $^1/_2$ teaspoon baking soda
- $^1/_2$ teaspoon salt
- 2   eggs, lightly beaten
- $^1/_3$ cup almond milk
- 2   tablespoons maple syrup
- 2   teaspoons coconut oil
- $1^1/_2$ teaspoons vanilla extract
- $^1/_2$ teaspoon finely shredded orange or lemon zest
- $^1/_2$ cup fresh blueberries, plus extra for garnish

INSTRUCTIONS

1 In a saucepan, cook sweet potato for 10 minutes or until tender in enough boiling water to cover; drain. In a medium bowl, mash sweet potato with a fork; set aside.
2 In a large bowl, stir together almond flour, coconut flour, cinnamon, nutmeg, baking soda and salt.
3 Add eggs to sweet potato. Whisk in almond milk, maple syrup, coconut oil, vanilla extract and orange or lemon zest. Gently stir in blueberries.
4 Lightly grease and preheat a waffle iron. Add batter to waffle iron according to manufacturer's directions. (Use a spatula to spread batter—it will be thick.) Close lid and do not open until waffles are done. Bake according to manufacturer's directions.
5 Remove waffles from pan and place on plates. Garnish with blueberries and maple syrup, honey or agave syrup, as desired.

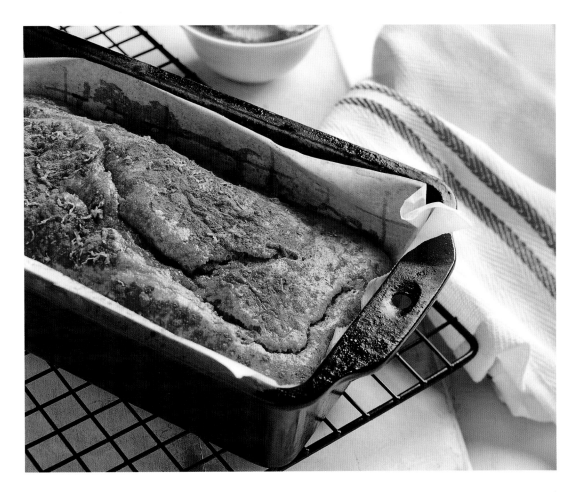

ON-THE-RUN BREAKFAST LOAF

Grab a slice of this quick bread on your
way out the door and stay satisfied all morning.

PREP 10 minutes
TOTAL 55 minutes–1 hour, 5 minutes
SERVINGS 6

INGREDIENTS

    Coconut oil
1 cup roasted almond butter
    (100 percent almonds)
4 eggs
4 tablespoons raw honey
¼ cup finely chopped raw coconut
2 tablespoons ground cinnamon
1 teaspoon finely shredded lemon zest
½ teaspoon baking soda
½ teaspoon sea salt
¼ teaspoon grated fresh nutmeg

INSTRUCTIONS

1 Preheat oven to 325°F. Grease an 8×4-inch loaf pan with coconut oil; line bottom and sides with parchment paper.

2 In a large bowl, beat almond butter with a mixer on medium until creamy. Beat in eggs, honey, coconut, cinnamon, lemon zest, baking soda, salt and nutmeg. Spread batter into prepared loaf pan.

3 Bake 25 minutes or until a toothpick inserted in center comes out clean. Cool in pan 10 minutes. Remove loaf from pan; cool on wire rack 10 to 20 minutes before slicing.

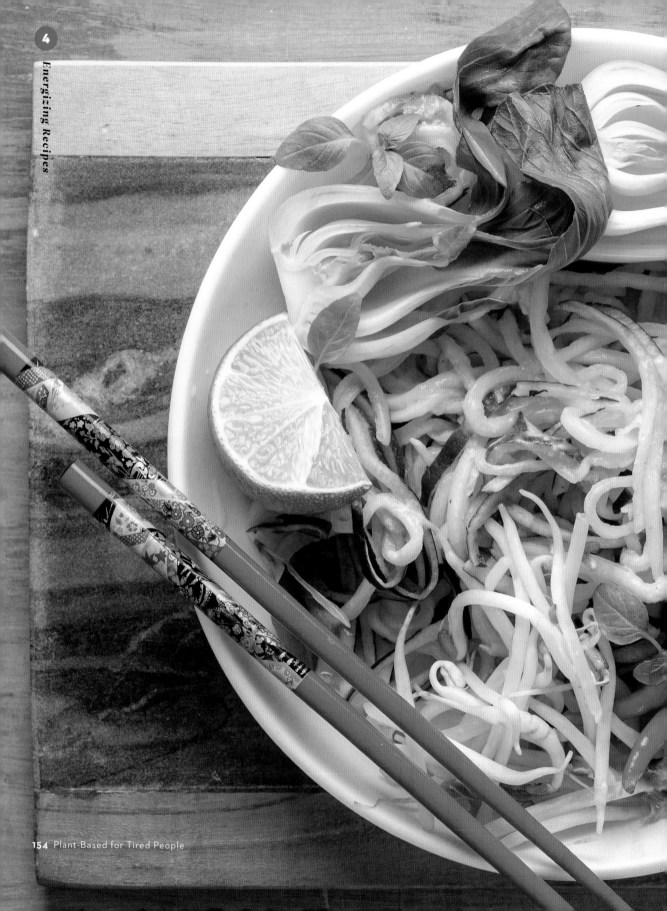

Salads, Sandwiches & Soups

PAD THAI ZOODLE SALAD

Spiralized veggies lighten up this dish, while traditional seasonings help give it an authentic flavor.

PREP 10 minutes
TOTAL 15 minutes
SERVINGS 4

INGREDIENTS

- 2/3 cup peanut butter
- 6 tablespoons sesame oil, divided
- 2 tablespoons lime juice
- 1 teaspoon salt
- 1/2 teaspoon red pepper flakes
- 2 (7-ounce) packages zucchini zoodles
- 4 heads baby bok choy, halved lengthwise
  Garnishes: bean sprouts, chopped peanuts, lime wedges, whole bird's-eye (Thai) chiles, Thai basil leaves

INSTRUCTIONS

1 To make dressing, in a small bowl, combine peanut butter, 4 tablespoons sesame oil, lime juice, salt and red pepper flakes until smooth. Set aside.

2 In a large skillet over medium-high heat, heat remaining sesame oil. Add zoodles and baby bok choy. Cook for 2 to 3 minutes.

3 Toss dressing with zoodles and bok choy. Divide evenly between four plates.

4 Garnish with bean sprouts, chopped peanuts, lime wedges, bird's-eye chiles and Thai basil leaves, as desired.

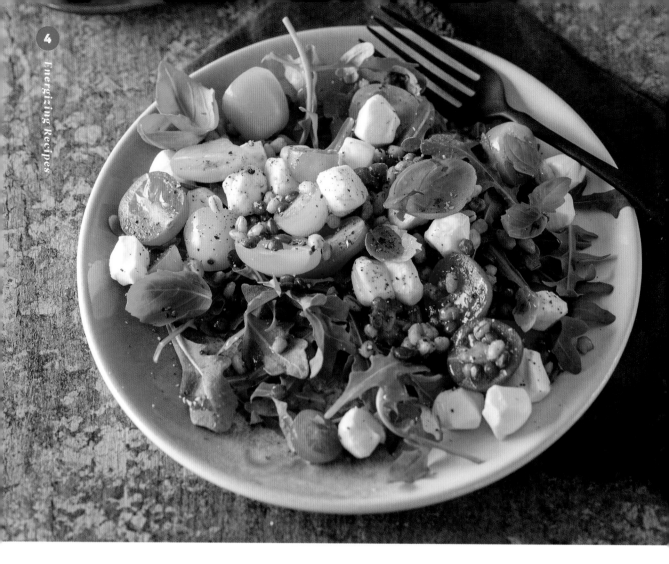

CAPRESE BARLEY AND GREEN LENTIL SALAD

Barley and lentils pair up together to pack a powerful nutrition punch that's high in fiber, protein, iron and selenium. Get the combo that comes as a microwavable version and you'll have this dish ready to go in just a few minutes.

PREP 5 minutes

TOTAL 10 minutes

SERVINGS 4

INGREDIENTS

- 1 (8.8-ounce) microwavable bag barley and green lentils, cooked according to package directions
- 1 pint multicolored cherry tomatoes, halved
- 1 (8-ounce) container pearl mozzarella, drained
- 1/4 cup olive oil
- 2 tablespoons red wine vinegar
- 1 tablespoon Dijon mustard
- 1/4 teaspoon sea salt
- 1/4 teaspoon ground black pepper
  Garnishes: basil leaves, micro radish greens

INSTRUCTIONS

1 In a large bowl, toss barley/lentil mixture, tomatoes and mozzarella.

2 To make dressing, in a blender, mix olive oil, red wine vinegar, mustard, salt and pepper until smooth.

3 Pour dressing over barley mixture; toss to combine.

4 Garnish as desired.

MEDITERRANEAN BULGUR SALAD

Bulgur is known as a plant-based protein that's high in iron, but it also has more fiber than quinoa, oats or millet. Because of its quick cooking time and mild flavor, it's ideal for those who are new to whole-grain cooking. In the Mediterranean, it's classically paired with cucumber, tomato and feta cheese.

PREP 20 minutes
TOTAL 2 hours, 30 minutes
SERVINGS 4

INGREDIENTS

SALAD

- 1 cup bulgur wheat
- 1 cup hot water
- 1 medium tomato, chopped
- 1/2 medium cucumber, seeded and chopped
- 1/2 medium red bell pepper, chopped
- 1 cup chopped fresh parsley
- 1/4 cup chopped fresh mint or cilantro
- 2 tablespoons sliced green onion
- 6 tablespoons crumbled feta cheese

DRESSING

- 2 tablespoons fresh lemon juice
- 2 tablespoons white wine vinegar
- 2 tablespoons olive oil
- 1 clove garlic, minced
- 1/4 teaspoon salt
- 1/4 teaspoon ground black pepper

INSTRUCTIONS

1 Place the bulgur wheat in a large bowl. Add hot water; let stand 30 minutes or until water is absorbed. If necessary, drain any excess water.

2 Meanwhile, to make dressing, in a small bowl, whisk together lemon juice, white wine vinegar, olive oil, garlic, salt and pepper. Set aside.

3 For salad, add tomato, cucumber, bell pepper, parsley, mint or cilantro, and green onion to bulgur. Drizzle with dressing; toss until coated and well combined. Top with feta. Cover and refrigerate 2 to 3 hours before serving.

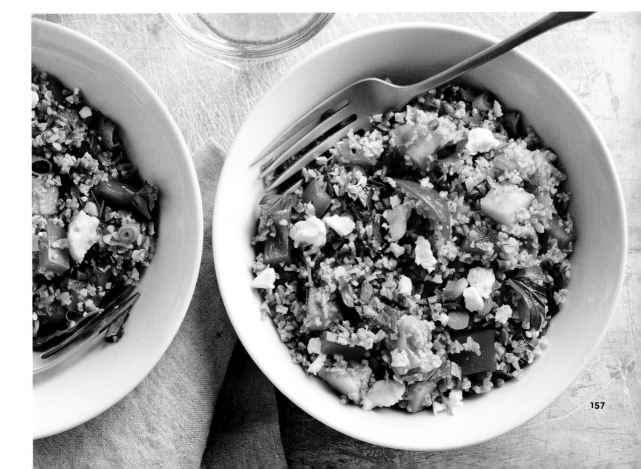

KALE CAESAR SALAD WITH GARLIC ROASTED CHICKPEAS

Raw or cooked, kale is the king of the supergreens. Tahini is full of good fats and may reduce inflammation.

PREP 5 minutes
TOTAL 15 minutes
SERVINGS 4

INGREDIENTS

- ½ cup olive oil
- 2 tablespoons lemon juice
- 2 tablespoons tahini
- 1 tablespoon Dijon mustard
- 1 teaspoon minced garlic
- ¼ teaspoon sea salt
- 1 (15-ounce) can chickpeas, drained and rinsed
- 1 teaspoon garlic salt
- 1 teaspoon ground black pepper
- 4 cups chopped kale leaves
  Garnish: lemon wedges

INSTRUCTIONS

1 To make dressing, in a blender, add olive oil, lemon juice, tahini, mustard, garlic and sea salt; blend until smooth. Set aside.
2 In a large skillet over medium heat, add chickpeas, garlic salt and pepper. Toast for 5 minutes or until chickpeas begin to dry out.
3 Divide kale evenly between four plates; drizzle with dressing and sprinkle with chickpeas.
4 Garnish with lemon wedges.

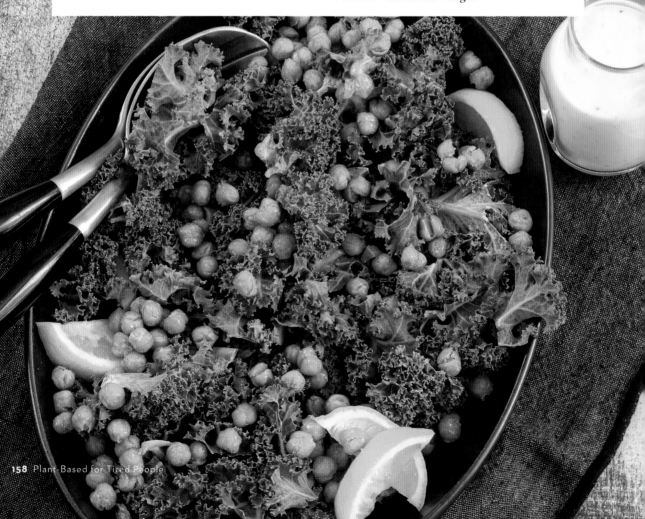

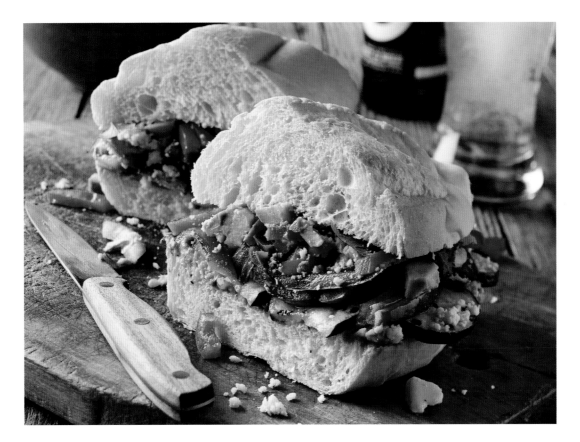

GRILLED VEGETABLE AND AVOCADO TORTAS

Tortas are a popular and tasty Mexican street food. Cut out the queso fresco to make it vegan.

PREP 35 minutes
TOTAL 40 minutes
SERVINGS 4

INGREDIENTS

- 1 tablespoon canola oil
- 1 cup sliced green bell pepper
- 1 cup sliced red bell pepper
- 1 cup sliced red onion
- 1 small zucchini, sliced
- ½ teaspoon salt
- ½ teaspoon ground black pepper
- 2 ripe avocados, pitted and diced
- 1 teaspoon hot green pepper sauce
- 4 teleras (Mexican-style soft sandwich rolls)
- ¼ cup crumbled queso fresco (optional)
- ¼ cup chopped fresh cilantro

INSTRUCTIONS

1 Preheat grill to medium-high heat for direct grilling. Drizzle oil over bell peppers, onion and zucchini; sprinkle with salt and black pepper. Place vegetables in a grill basket. Grill vegetables, uncovered, directly over heat 6 to 8 minutes or to desired doneness. Remove from grill.

2 To assemble tortas, in a small bowl, mash half of the diced avocados with hot pepper sauce. Spread avocado mixture onto bottom halves of rolls. Layer grilled vegetables and queso (optional) on mashed avocado. Top with remaining diced avocado and cilantro. Top with upper halves of rolls, pressing down firmly.

3 Tightly wrap tortas in plastic wrap; refrigerate until ready to serve. To serve, unwrap and cut each torta in half.

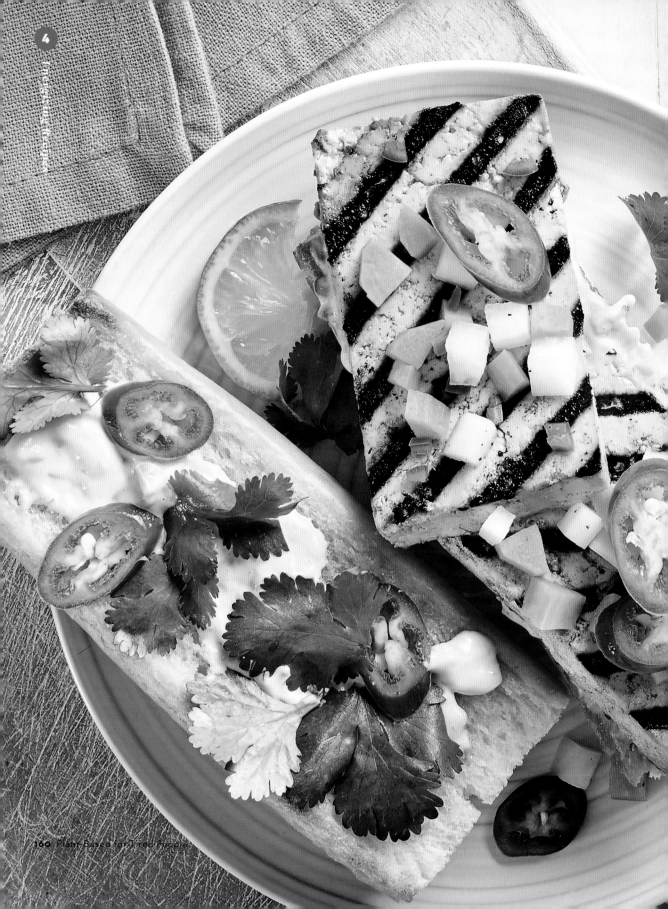

VEGETARIAN BÁNH MÌ

Bánh mì is Vietnamese for bread. But today you'll find that it refers to a Vietnamese-inspired sandwich with pickled vegetables. Instead of pork, chicken or other meat, we used extra-firm tofu and topped it with a 15-minute-brined pickled vegetable mixture.

PREP 45 minutes
TOTAL 1 hour, 35 minutes
SERVINGS 2

INGREDIENTS

PICKLED VEGETABLES
- ¼ cup finely chopped carrot
- ¼ cup finely chopped daikon radish
- ¼ cup finely chopped cucumber
- ½ small jalapeño pepper, seeded and finely chopped (optional)
- ½ cup warm water
- ¼ cup rice wine vinegar
- 1 tablespoon sugar
- 1 teaspoon salt
- ¼ teaspoon ground black pepper

SRIRACHA MAYONNAISE
- 2 tablespoons mayonnaise
- 1 teaspoon Sriracha sauce

SANDWICHES
- 8 ounce block extra-firm tofu
- ½ teaspoon finely shredded lime peel
- 1 tablespoon fresh lime juice
- 1 tablespoon honey
- 1 tablespoon soy sauce
- 1 clove garlic, minced
- Canola oil
- ½ French baguette, split and toasted
- Chopped fresh cilantro and/or seeded sliced jalapeño pepper (optional)

INSTRUCTIONS

1 For pickled vegetables, in a 16-ounce jar, combine carrot, daikon radish, cucumber and jalapeño (if desired). In a small bowl, combine warm water, rice wine vinegar, sugar, salt and black pepper. Stir until sugar and salt are dissolved. Pour mixture over vegetables in jar. Cover and refrigerate at least 15 minutes (or up to 1 week).

2 For Sriracha mayonnaise, in a prep dish or custard cup, combine mayonnaise and Sriracha sauce; cover and refrigerate until serving.

3 For sandwiches, drain tofu at least 15 minutes before serving, pressing occasionally to squeeze out excess liquid. Cut tofu into 4 slices; place in a medium resealable plastic bag. Combine lime peel and juice, honey, soy sauce and garlic. Pour lime marinade over tofu; close bag to seal. Turn bag to evenly coat tofu with marinade. Let stand at room temperature 15 minutes.

4 Lightly oil a cold grill pan or heavy skillet. Preheat over medium-high heat. Remove tofu from marinade; discard marinade. Cook tofu in heated grill pan 5 minutes or until heated through and slightly golden, turning once.

5 To assemble sandwiches, cut baguette crosswise in half. Spread Sriracha mayonnaise on cut sides of bottoms and tops. Place tofu and pickled vegetables on baguette bottoms. Top with cilantro and sliced jalapeño, if desired. Top with remaining baguette halves.

HUMMUS WRAPS WITH GRILLED VEGGIES

In the summer, when fresh produce is at its peak, take advantage of the sweet tastes of just-picked veggies by searing and tucking them into tortillas with hummus.

PREP 20 minutes
TOTAL 40 minutes
SERVINGS 2

INGREDIENTS

- 2 $1/2$-inch-thick slices red onion
- 1 small yellow bell pepper, quartered
- $1/2$ small eggplant, cut into $1/2$-inch-thick slices
- 3 teaspoons olive oil, divided
- 2 tablespoons chopped fresh basil
- $1/8$ teaspoon salt
- $1/2$ cup garlic hummus
- 2 8-inch sun-dried tomato-basil tortillas
- $1/4$ cup crumbled goat cheese

INSTRUCTIONS

1 Preheat a grill pan or large cast-iron skillet over medium-high heat. Brush onion, bell pepper and eggplant with $1^{1}/_{2}$ teaspoons olive oil. Add onion and bell pepper to heated grill pan; cook 6 minutes or until grill marks appear, turning once. Transfer vegetables to a cutting board.

2 Add eggplant to grill pan; cook 6 minutes or until grill marks appear, turning once. Transfer to the cutting board. Coarsely chop vegetables. Drizzle with remaining $1^{1}/_{2}$ teaspoons olive oil; sprinkle with basil and salt. Toss to combine.

3 To assemble, spread $1/4$ cup hummus on each tortilla, leaving a $1/2$-inch border around edges. Spoon half of vegetables on top of hummus just below the center of each tortilla; sprinkle each with half of the goat cheese. Fold bottoms of tortillas up and over filling. Fold in sides; roll up. Cut diagonally in half to serve.

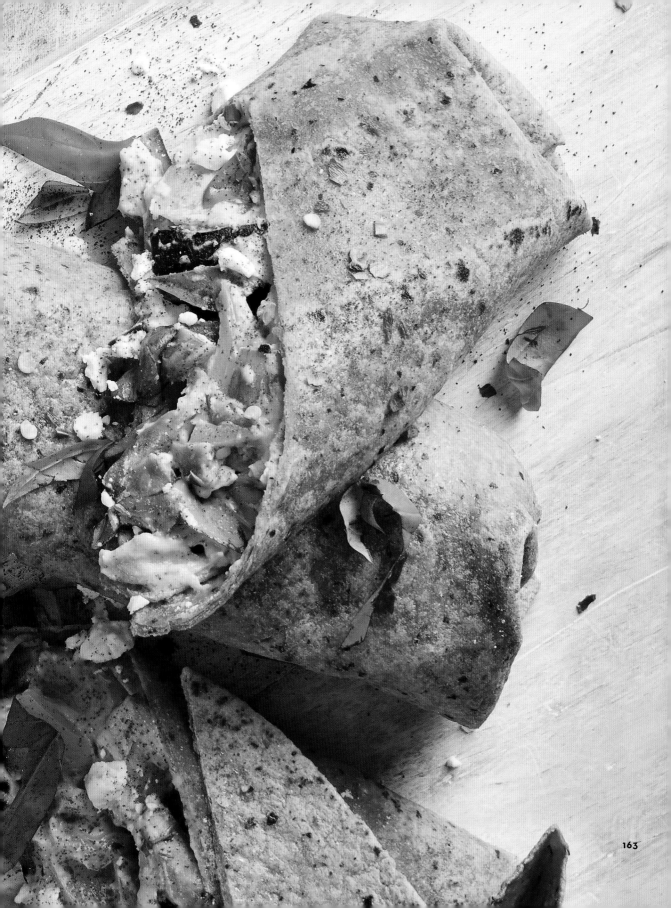

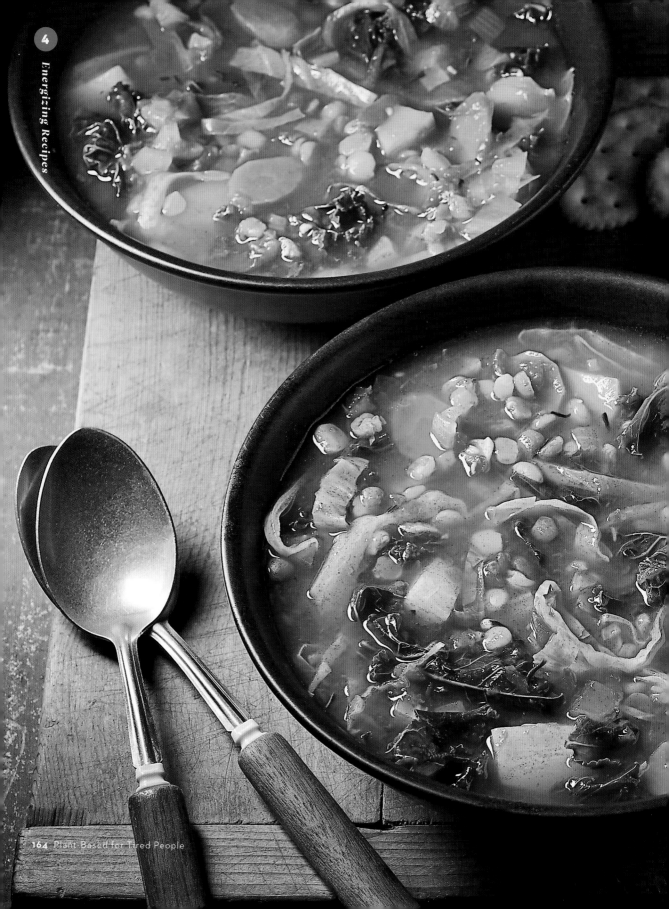

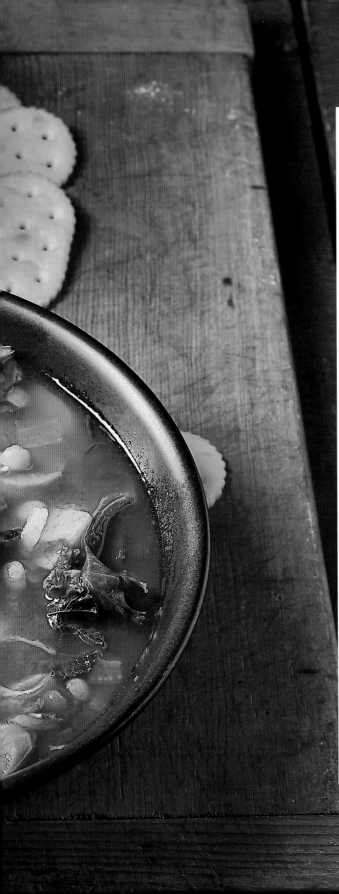

MIXED SPLIT PEA SOUP WITH GREENS

Kale adds a vitamin boost to this colorful mix of split peas, and a generous amount of garlic gives it an addictive aroma.

PREP 10 minutes
TOTAL 2 hours, 15 minutes
SERVINGS 8

INGREDIENTS

- 3 tablespoons extra-virgin olive oil
- 1 large onion, chopped
- 2 medium carrots, peeled and sliced
- 2 medium parsnips, peeled and sliced
- 2 ribs celery, chopped
  Salt and ground black pepper
- 4 cloves garlic, minced
- ¾ cup yellow split peas
- ¾ cup green split peas
- 1 (28-ounce) can crushed tomatoes
- ¼ small head green cabbage, finely shredded
- 3 cups torn kale
- 3 bay leaves
- 1 teaspoon dried savory

INSTRUCTIONS

1 In a large, heavy-bottomed pot or Dutch oven, heat olive oil. Add onion, carrots, parsnips and celery and cook over medium-low heat, stirring occasionally, until softened, about 6 minutes. Season with generous pinches of salt and pepper. Add garlic and cook, stirring, another minute or until fragrant.

2 Add split peas, tomatoes and enough water to cover; bring to a boil. Add cabbage, kale, bay leaves, savory and enough water to cover by 2 inches. Bring to a boil, reduce heat to low and simmer, covered, 2 hours. Stir every 20 minutes and add water as necessary. Salt and pepper to taste and serve once peas are soft and soup has reached desired consistency.

BARLEY, BEAN & LENTIL SOUP

Barley adds nutty flavor, fiber and plenty of vitamins to this comforting mix.

PREP 10 minutes
TOTAL 1 hour, 10 minutes
SERVINGS 4 to 6

INGREDIENTS

- 1 tablespoon olive oil
- 1 white or yellow onion, chopped
- 2 stalks celery, with leaves, chopped
- 2 carrots, chopped
- 2 cloves garlic, minced
- 2 tablespoons tomato paste
- 1 teaspoon dried oregano
- 1 teaspoon dried basil
- 2 teaspoons salt
- 1 teaspoon ground black pepper
- ½ cup barley
- ⅓ cup lentils
- 2 Yukon Gold potatoes, quartered
- 1 (15-ounce) can red kidney beans, drained and rinsed
- 2 tablespoons chopped parsley (optional)

INSTRUCTIONS

1 In a large soup pot, heat olive oil over medium heat. Add onion, celery, carrots and garlic. Cook until vegetables begin to soften and become fragrant, about 3 to 5 minutes. Stir in tomato paste, oregano, basil, salt and pepper. Sauté 3 to 5 minutes, stirring frequently.
2 Add barley, lentils, potatoes and kidney beans; stir to combine. Add enough water to pot to cover contents by about 2 inches. Stir to combine, cover partially and simmer about 1 hour. Remove soup from heat; let sit for a few minutes before serving.
3 Top with parsley just before serving, if desired.

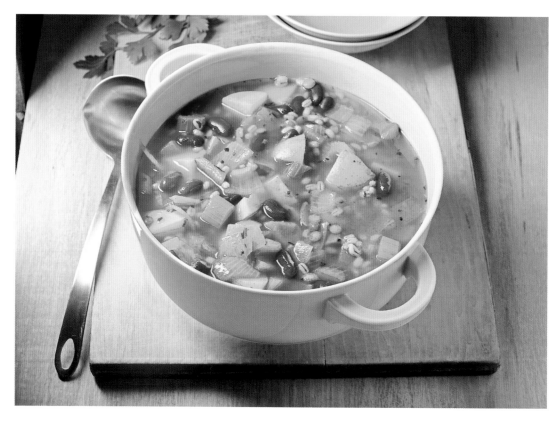

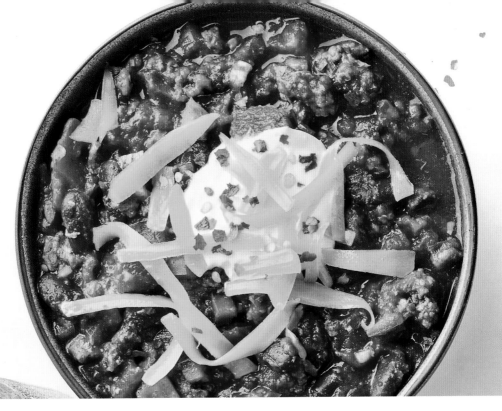

SPICY TWO-BEAN VEGGIE CHILI

This meatless chili is based on beans and a wide variety of veggies. Leave off the cheese and sour cream to make it dairy-free and vegan friendly.

PREP 40 minutes
TOTAL 1 hour, 15 minutes
SERVINGS 4

INGREDIENTS

- 2 tablespoons vegetable oil
- 1 medium yellow onion, finely chopped
- 1 medium red bell pepper, finely chopped
- 1 large carrot, chopped
- 1 large stalk celery, finely chopped
- 1 small serrano chile, seeded and finely chopped
- 4 cloves garlic, minced
- 3 tablespoons chili powder
- 2 tablespoons finely chopped fresh cilantro
- 2 teaspoons ground cumin
- 1 teaspoon sugar
- 1 teaspoon smoked paprika
- 1 teaspoon dried Mexican oregano
- 1/4 teaspoon ground cinnamon
- 1/2 teaspoon salt
- 1/4 teaspoon ground black pepper
- 1 28-ounce can diced fire-roasted tomatoes, undrained
- 1/4 cup tomato paste
- 1 15-ounce can pinto or black beans, drained and rinsed
- 1 15-ounce can red kidney beans, drained and rinsed
  Toppings: shredded cheddar cheese, sour cream, crushed red pepper (optional)

INSTRUCTIONS

1 In a 4-quart saucepan or Dutch oven, heat vegetable oil over medium heat. Add onion; cook and stir 6 minutes or until tender.

2 Add red bell pepper, carrot, celery, serrano chile and garlic. Cook 5 minutes, stirring often. Stir in chili powder, cilantro, cumin, sugar, smoked paprika, Mexican oregano, cinnamon, salt and black pepper. Cook 1 minute.

3 Stir in undrained tomatoes, tomato paste and pinto (or black) and red kidney beans. Bring to a boil. Reduce heat to medium-low. Gently simmer, uncovered, for at least 30 minutes or for up to 2 hours to blend flavors.

4 Ladle chili into 4 bowls. Add toppings, if desired.

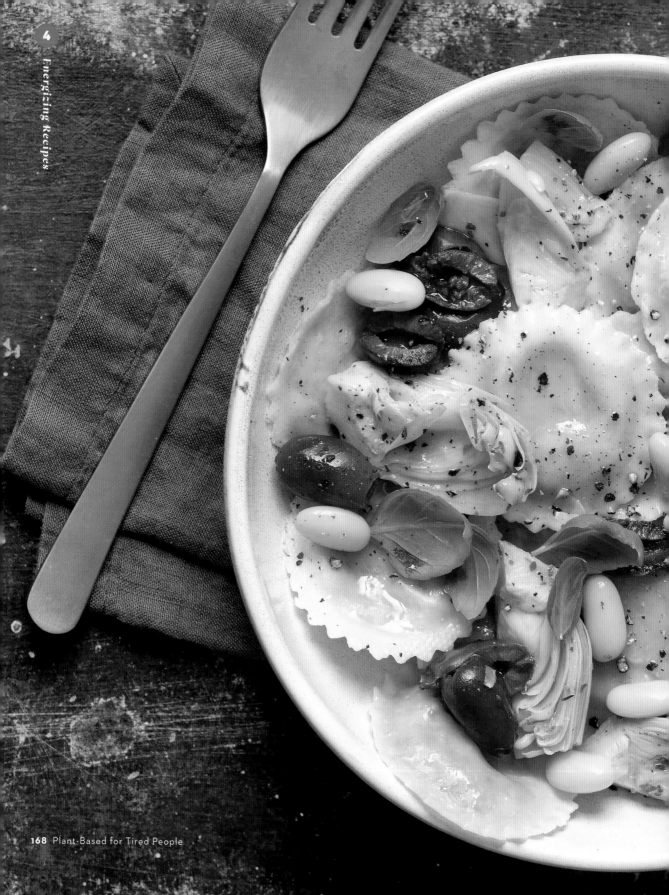

Delicious Dinners

SPINACH RAVIOLI WITH ARTICHOKES AND OLIVES

Artichokes are packed with fiber and have more protein than the average veggie, to boot! The jarred hearts are usually marinated in olive oil and lemon or vinegar, so drain them well before using so the flavor doesn't overwhelm the dish.

PREP 10 minutes
TOTAL 20 minutes
SERVINGS 4

INGREDIENTS

- 1 (8-ounce) package refrigerated spinach-filled ravioli
- 1/4 cup olive oil
- 1/2 teaspoon salt
- 1/2 teaspoon ground black pepper
- 1 teaspoon chopped garlic
- 1 (12-ounce) jar artichoke hearts, drained
- 1/2 cup kalamata olives, drained and halved
- 1 (15-ounce) can cannellini beans, drained and rinsed
- Garnish: basil leaves

INSTRUCTIONS

1 Cook ravioli according to package directions. Drain; set aside and keep warm.
2 Meanwhile, in a small bowl, mix olive oil, salt, pepper and garlic.
3 In a large bowl, combine ravioli, artichoke hearts, kalamata olives and cannellini beans. Drizzle with olive oil mixture; garnish with basil leaves.

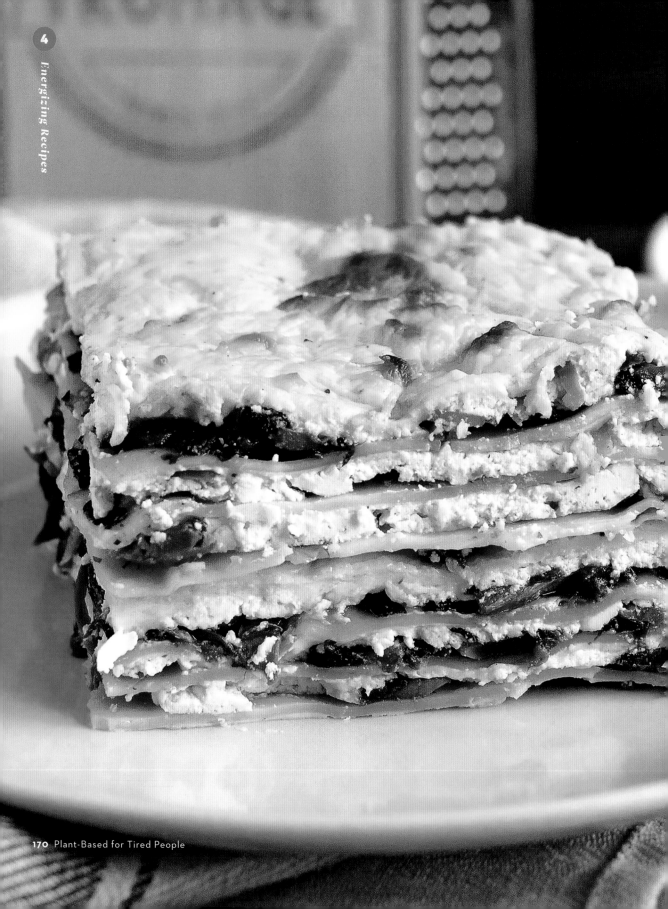

MUSHROOM LASAGNA WITH SWISS CHARD AND RICOTTA

Swiss chard is similar to spinach, although slightly sweeter and not as tender.

PREP 40 minutes
TOTAL 1 hour, 45 minutes
SERVINGS 8

INGREDIENTS

- 6 tablespoons butter
- 1/2 cup all-purpose flour
- 3 1/2 cups hot whole milk
  Sea salt and ground black pepper
- 1/2 teaspoon ground nutmeg, divided
- 6 tablespoons olive oil, divided
- 1 medium red onion, chopped
- 1 pound baby portobello mushrooms, sliced
- 4 cloves garlic, minced
- 1 pound Swiss chard, center rib and stem cut from each leaf, chopped
  Zest of one lemon
- 12 dried lasagna noodles
- 2 tablespoons olive oil
- 1 (15-ounce) container whole-milk ricotta cheese
- 1 cup fontina cheese, grated
- 1 cup Parmigiano-Reggiano, grated

INSTRUCTIONS

1 To make béchamel sauce, in a saucepan, melt butter with flour over low heat, whisking constantly to make the roux (paste). Slowly add half the hot milk to the roux; continue to whisk constantly. Add remaining milk slowly while stirring until it comes to a boil. Season with salt, black pepper and 1/4 teaspoon nutmeg; continue stirring until consistency is smooth. If any lumps form, beat them out rapidly with the whisk until they dissolve. Remove from heat and set aside.

2 In a large skillet over medium-high heat, heat 2 tablespoons olive oil. Add onion, mushrooms and garlic. Sauté until onion is tender, and mushrooms and garlic are golden, about 7 to 8 minutes. Mix in remaining 1/4 teaspoon nutmeg; season with salt and pepper. Add chard, lower heat to medium, and cover until the chard wilts, about 3 to 4 minutes, stirring occasionally. Stir in lemon zest.

3 Preheat oven to 350°F. Meanwhile, in a large pot of boiling salted water, cook noodles according to package directions until tender but firm, stirring occasionally. Drain; arrange in single layer on a sheet of plastic wrap. Brush a 13×9-inch glass or stainless steel baking dish with olive oil to coat. Spread a quarter of the béchamel in dish. Add a layer of 4 lasagna noodles, spaced evenly so they don't overlap. Spread half of chard/mushroom mixture over pasta. Drop half the ricotta in dollops and spread. Sprinkle with half the fontina, then half the Parmigiano-Reggiano. Repeat layering with noodles, chard and mushrooms, ricotta, fontina, Parmigiano-Reggiano, béchamel and noodles.

4 Cook in bottom of oven for 30 minutes, then move to middle of oven, raise temperature to 375°F and cook another 15 minutes until golden and crispy all over. Let rest for 15 minutes before serving.

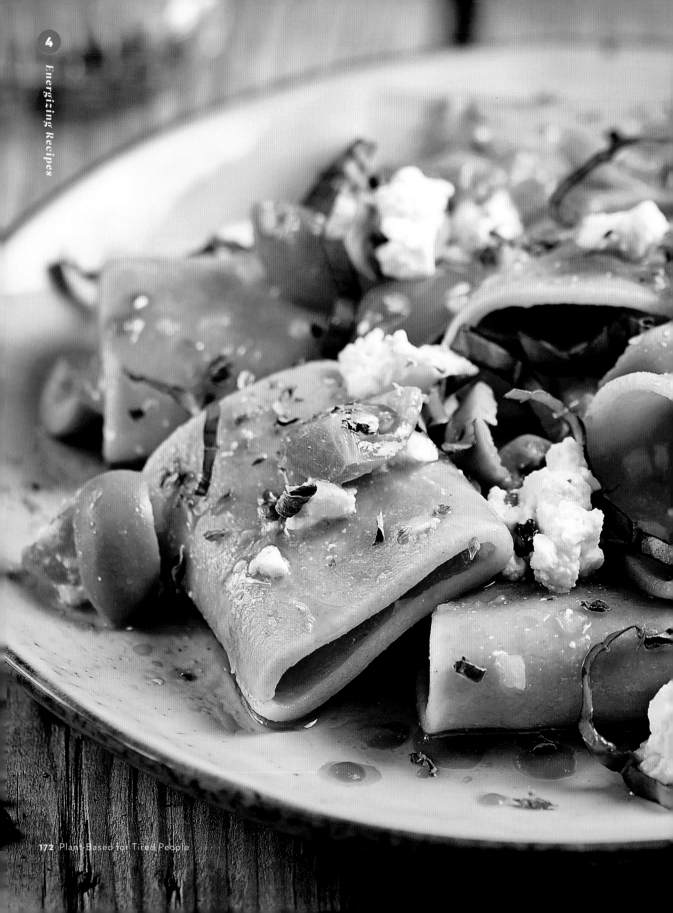

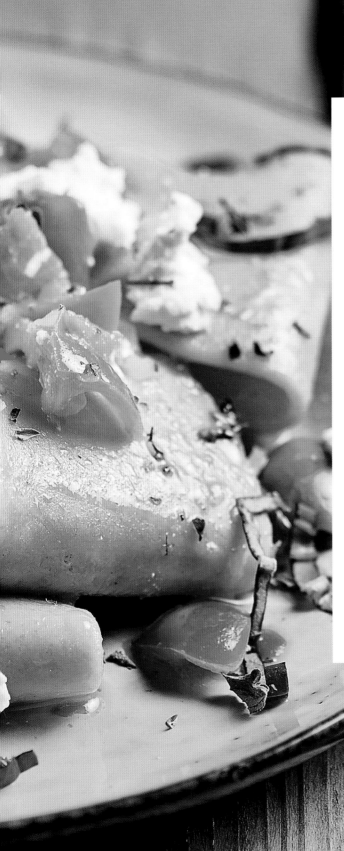

WHOLE-WHEAT PASTA WITH OLIVES, ROASTED CHERRY TOMATOES AND RICOTTA

With its nutty flavor, whole-wheat pasta tastes best served with bold ingredients.

PREP 10 minutes
TOTAL 25 minutes
SERVINGS 4–6

INGREDIENTS

25 to 30 cherry tomatoes
Olive oil
Sea salt to taste
1 teaspoon dried basil
1 teaspoon dried oregano
1 pound dried whole-wheat rigatoni
1/2 cup fresh ricotta
1 1/2 tablespoons fresh basil, chiffonade
1/3 cup grated Parmigiano-Reggiano
1 cup green olives, pitted and halved

INSTRUCTIONS

1 Preheat oven to 350°F. Wash and dry tomatoes. Cut in half and place on a cookie sheet lined with parchment paper. Drizzle with olive oil and sprinkle with salt, dried basil and oregano. Roast for 15 minutes.
2 Meanwhile, cook pasta in boiling salted water according to package directions. In a medium bowl, mix ricotta, fresh basil and Parmigiano-Reggiano.
3 Chop tomatoes coarsely. When pasta is done, drain; top with tomatoes, cheese and basil mixture, and olives. Drizzle with olive oil and toss to coat.

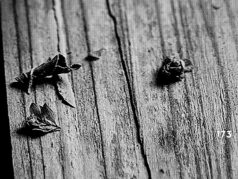

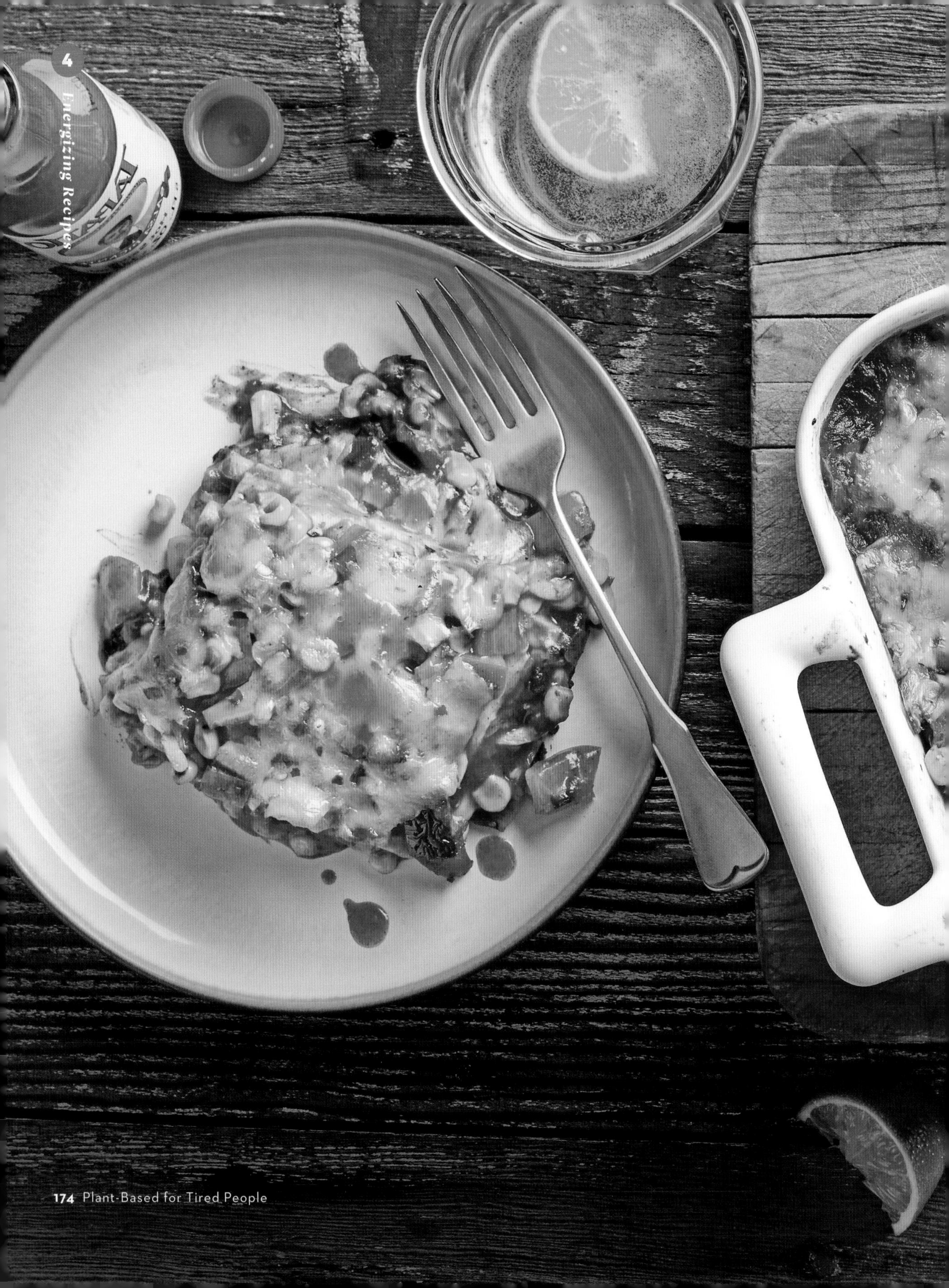

MEXICAN PEPPER, BLACK BEAN AND CORN CASSEROLE

Black beans and an assortment of pan-roasted vegetables keep this meatless casserole on the healthier side.

PREP 1 hour
TOTAL 1 hour, 35 minutes
SERVINGS 12

INGREDIENTS

- 1   tablespoon olive oil
- 1   small red onion, chopped
- 2   yellow bell peppers, chopped
- 1   green bell pepper, chopped
- 1   medium poblano chile, seeded and chopped
- 2   teaspoons chili powder, divided
- 2   teaspoons ground cumin, divided
- 1/4 teaspoon cayenne pepper
- 2   cups frozen whole-kernel corn
- 1   teaspoon salt
- 1/4 teaspoon ground black pepper
- 18 6-inch white corn tortillas
- 1   16-ounce can refried black beans
- 2   cups red enchilada sauce
- 2   cups shredded pepper Jack cheese
      Toppings: fresh chopped cilantro, guacamole, sour cream

INSTRUCTIONS

1 To pan-roast vegetables, heat oil in large skillet over medium heat. Add onion, bell peppers and poblano chile. Sprinkle with 1 teaspoon chili powder, 1 teaspoon cumin and cayenne pepper. Cook until slightly charred, stirring occasionally. Transfer vegetables to a plate.

2 In same skillet, pan-roast corn with remaining 1 teaspoon chili powder and 1 teaspoon cumin. Transfer to plate with the other vegetables; sprinkle with salt and pepper.

3 Preheat oven to 400°F. Grease a 13×9-inch baking dish. Cut the tortillas into narrow strips; set aside. In a bowl, combine refried beans with enough water to get them to a spreadable consistency.

4 To assemble, spread thin layer of refried beans in the bottom of the baking dish. On the beans, layer half the tortilla strips, all of the remaining refried beans, half of vegetable mix, half the enchilada sauce and half the cheese. Repeat layers with remaining tortilla strips, vegetables, sauce and cheese.

5 Cover dish with foil. Bake 15 to 20 minutes or until heated through and cheese is melted. Serve with cilantro, guacamole and sour cream on the side.

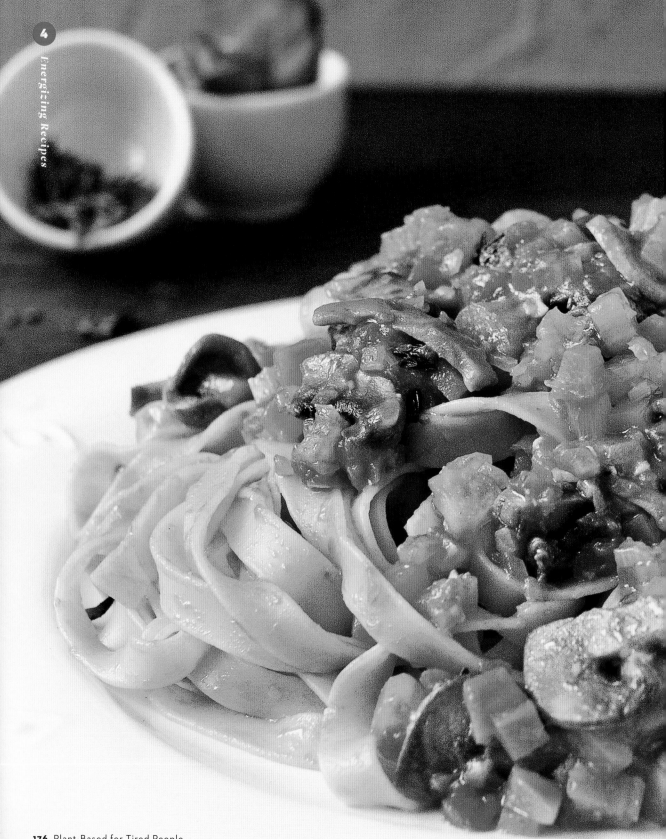

FETTUCCINE WITH VEGETARIAN MUSHROOM BOLOGNESE

It's so hearty, you won't miss the meat!

PREP 15 minutes
TOTAL 1 hour
SERVINGS 4-6

INGREDIENTS

- ¹/₃ cup dried porcini mushrooms (or 1 cup frozen)
- 3 tablespoon olive oil, divided
- 8 ounces baby portobellos, finely diced
  Sea salt
- 1 large yellow onion, chopped
- 4 cloves garlic, minced
- 2 medium carrots, finely diced
- 2 celery stalks, finely diced
- 1 teaspoon fresh thyme
- 2 tablespoons tomato paste
- 1 (28-ounce) can whole peeled tomatoes, undrained
- 1 pound dried fettuccine or tagliatelle pasta
- ¹/₄ cup fresh basil, torn by hand

INSTRUCTIONS

1 If using dried mushrooms, place in a bowl and cover with boiling water; let soak 10 to 15 minutes.

2 In a large nonstick skillet over medium-high heat, heat 2 tablespoons olive oil. Add baby portobellos and a pinch of salt and sauté, stirring, until mushrooms begin to soften, about 5 to 8 minutes. Keep cooking until all the moisture has disappeared and mushrooms are golden brown, about 2 to 3 minutes. Transfer mushrooms to a bowl, then add onion, garlic, carrots and celery with remaining 1 tablespoon of olive oil and stir well. Cover and cook for 10 minutes, stirring often.

3 Add thyme and tomato paste. Drain porcini mushrooms, reserving the liquid; chop well and add to sauce, along with reserved liquid. Add cooked portobellos. Then add whole peeled tomatoes and juice, using a wooden spoon to break up tomatoes. Bring to a simmer; cook for 30 minutes until sauce thickens.

4 Meanwhile, in a large pot of boiling salted water, cook pasta according to package directions. Drain and toss with sauce, being sure to coat all the pasta. Stir in the basil just before serving.

ROASTED VEGETABLE AND CAULIFLOWER RICE BOWL

With a rainbow of roasted veggies, this bowl is as healthy as it is colorful.

PREP 15 minutes
TOTAL 25 minutes
SERVINGS 2

INGREDIENTS

- 1 orange bell pepper, coarsely chopped
- 1 red onion, sliced
- 1 pound Brussels sprouts, trimmed and halved
- 1 tablespoon olive oil
- ½ teaspoon sea salt
- ½ teaspoon ground black pepper
- ¼ cup olive oil
- 2 tablespoons Champagne vinegar
- 1 teaspoon Dijon mustard
- 1 (16-ounce) microwavable bag cauliflower rice, cooked according to package directions
  Garnish: micro parsley leaves

INSTRUCTIONS

1 Preheat oven to 425°F.
2 On a rimmed sheet pan, add pepper, onion and Brussels sprouts.
3 Drizzle with 1 tablespoon olive oil; sprinkle with salt and pepper.
4 Roast for 10 minutes, turning halfway through cooking. Remove from oven.
5 Meanwhile, to make dressing, in a small bowl, whisk together olive oil, vinegar and mustard until smooth.
6 Divide cooked cauliflower rice between two serving bowls.
7 Top evenly with roasted vegetables; drizzle with dressing.
8 Garnish with micro parsley leaves as desired.

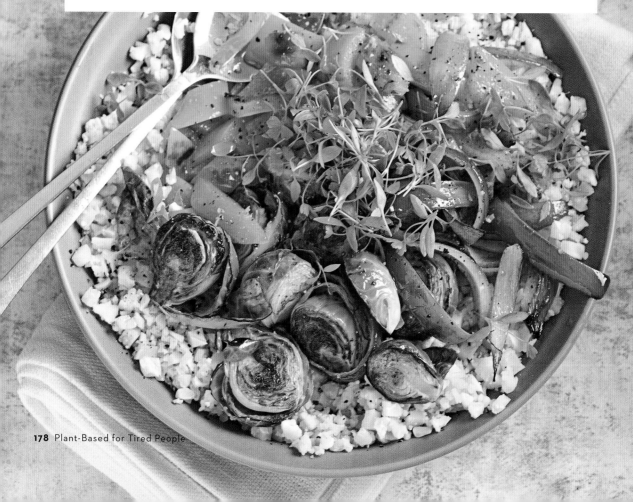

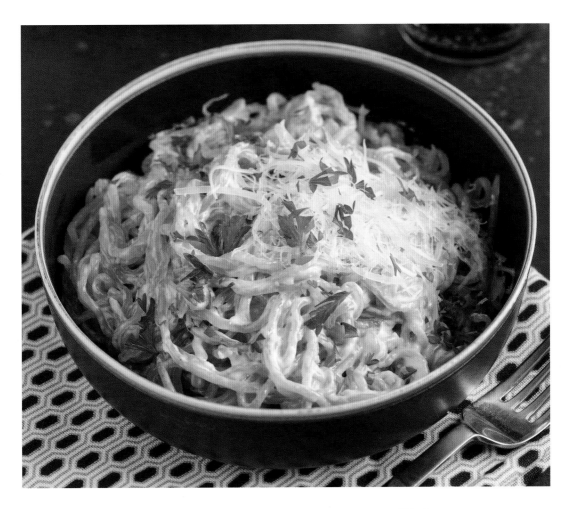

SPINACH "PASTA" ALFREDO

This rich and creamy dish will become a family favorite. You can also make it with zoodles.

PREP 5 minutes
TOTAL 15 minutes
SERVINGS 4

INGREDIENTS

- $1/2$ cup butter
- 2 cloves garlic, minced
- 2 cups heavy cream
- 4 ounces cream cheese, softened
- $1^1/2$ cups grated Parmesan cheese
- $1/4$ teaspoon nutmeg
- $1/4$ teaspoon salt
- $1/4$ teaspoon ground black pepper
- 2 (7-ounce) bags spinach shirataki pasta (Miracle Noodle), drained and rinsed
  Garnishes: cracked black pepper, chopped parsley, grated Parmesan

INSTRUCTIONS

1 In a Dutch oven over medium–high heat, melt butter. Add garlic and cook 2 minutes. Stir in cream and cream cheese until smooth.

2 Slowly stir in Parmesan cheese until well-incorporated and sauce thickens, about 5 minutes. Stir in nutmeg, salt, pepper and noodles.

3 Serve immediately with cracked black pepper, parsley and grated Parmesan on the side.

CHICKPEA AND SPELT BOWL WITH ROASTED BROCCOLI AND SHALLOTS

Spelt is an ancient grain. It is an excellent source of dietary fiber, and is also rich in iron, magnesium, phosphorus and zinc.

PREP 15 minutes
TOTAL 25 minutes
SERVINGS 2

INGREDIENTS

- 1 cup broccoli florets
- 2 shallots, quartered
- 1 cup cubed butternut squash
- 1 tablespoon avocado oil or olive oil
- ½ teaspoon sea salt
- ½ teaspoon ground black pepper
- 1 (8-ounce) package microwavable spelt, green lentils and long-grain brown rice, cooked according to package directions
- 1 (15.5-ounce) can chickpeas, drained and rinsed

INSTRUCTIONS

1 Preheat oven to 400°F.
2 On a rimmed sheet pan, place broccoli florets, shallots and squash. Drizzle with avocado oil or olive oil; sprinkle with salt and pepper.
3 Roast in oven for 10 minutes or until vegetables are browned, flipping halfway through cooking. Remove from oven.
4 Divide spelt, green lentils and brown rice mix between two individual serving bowls.
5 Top each bowl with roasted vegetables and chickpeas.

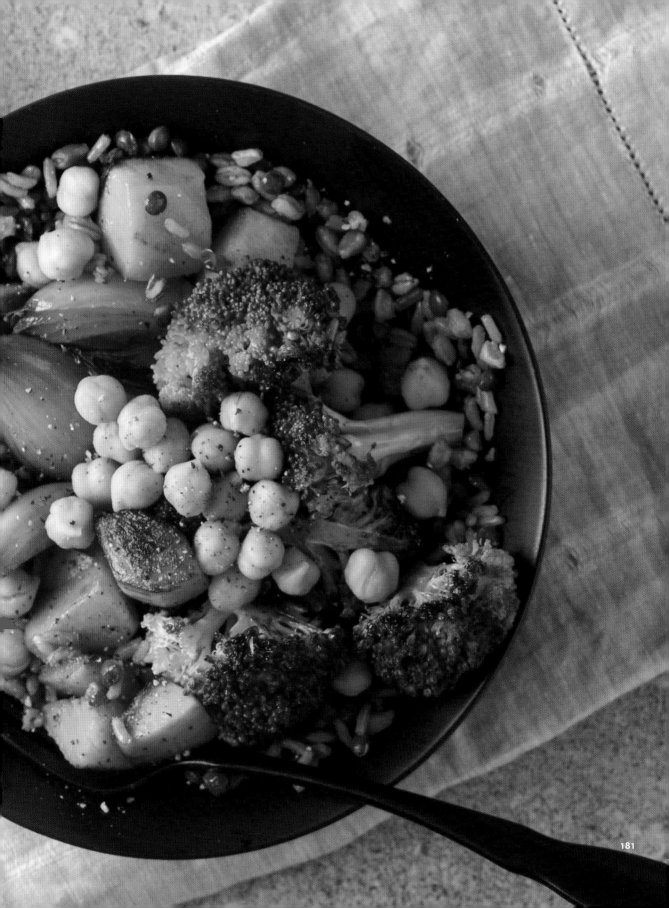

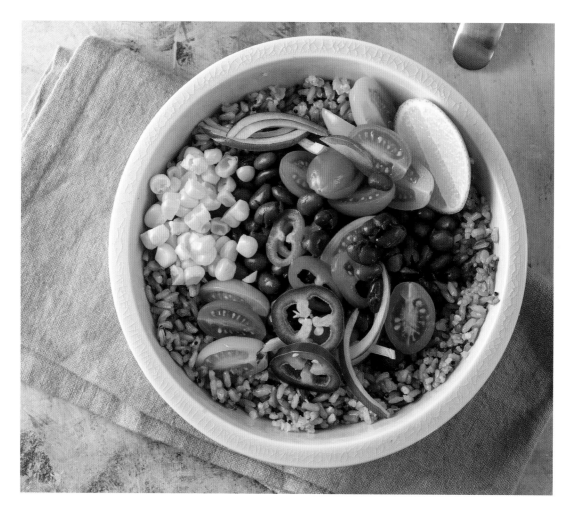

MEXICAN GRAIN BOWL WITH RED BEANS, CORN AND TOMATOES

Quinoa blends well with other grains like brown and red rice for a fiber-rich, high-protein base.

PREP 15 minutes
TOTAL 15 minutes
SERVINGS 2

INGREDIENTS

- 1 (8.5-ounce) bag microwavable organic quinoa, brown and red rice with flaxseed, cooked according to package directions
- ½ teaspoon sea salt
- ¼ teaspoon ground black pepper
- 1 (15-ounce) can red beans, drained and rinsed
- 1 pint cherry tomatoes, halved
- 1 ear of corn, scraped
- 1 small red onion, sliced
  Garnishes: jalapeño pepper slices, Fresno pepper slices, lime slices

INSTRUCTIONS

1 In a medium bowl, mix cooked quinoa and rice mixture, salt and pepper. Divide mixture between two individual serving bowls.
2 Evenly divide beans, tomatoes, corn and onion slices between serving bowls.
3 Serve with garnishes on the side.

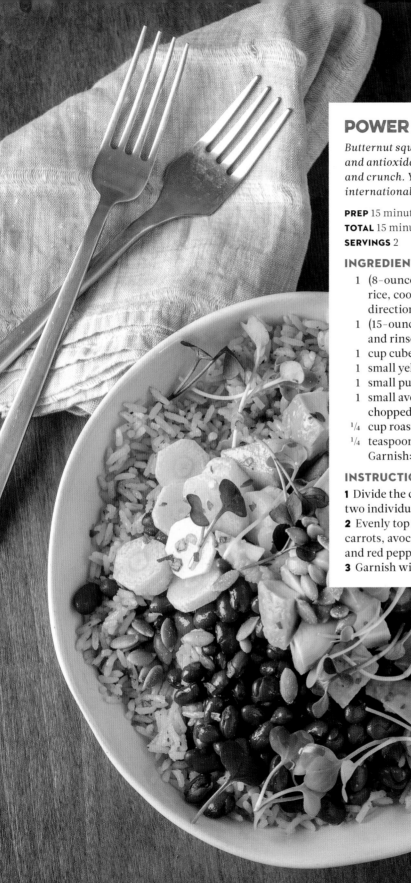

POWER BOWL

Butternut squash is full of vitamins, minerals and antioxidants while carrots add color and crunch. You can find turmeric rice in the international aisle at many grocery stores.

PREP 15 minutes
TOTAL 15 minutes
SERVINGS 2

INGREDIENTS

- 1 (8-ounce) microwavable bag turmeric rice, cooked according to package directions
- 1 (15-ounce) can black beans, drained and rinsed
- 1 cup cubed and cooked butternut squash
- 1 small yellow carrot, sliced
- 1 small purple carrot, sliced
- 1 small avocado, pitted and coarsely chopped
- 1/4 cup roasted pepitas or pumpkin seeds
- 1/4 teaspoon red pepper flakes
  Garnish: micro radish greens

INSTRUCTIONS

1 Divide the cooked turmeric rice between two individual serving bowls.
2 Evenly top with black beans, squash, carrots, avocado, pepitas or pumpkin seeds and red pepper flakes.
3 Garnish with micro radish greens.

VEGGIE TACOS WITH CHIPOTLE CREAM SAUCE

Chili-spiced lentils and oven-roasted cauliflower take center stage in these flavorful tacos.

PREP 30 minutes
TOTAL 1 hour, 30 minutes
SERVINGS 4

INGREDIENTS

SAVORY LENTILS

- 1 tablespoon olive oil
- 1 cup chopped yellow or white onion
- 2 medium shallots, minced
- 2 tablespoons tomato paste
- 1/2 teaspoon garlic powder
- 1/2 teaspoon ground cumin
- 1/2 teaspoon chili powder
- 2 cups vegetable broth
- 3/4 cup dried brown lentils, rinsed and drained

ROASTED CAULIFLOWER

- 1 large head cauliflower, cut into bite-size florets
- 3 tablespoons olive oil
- 1/2 teaspoon salt
- 1/4 teaspoon ground black pepper
- 1/8 teaspoon cayenne pepper

CHIPOTLE CREAM SAUCE

- 1/3 cup mayonnaise
- 1/2 teaspoon finely shredded lime peel
- 2 tablespoons fresh lime juice

- 2 tablespoons adobo sauce (from canned chipotle peppers) or chipotle hot sauce, to taste
  Salt and ground black pepper

TACOS

- 8 6-inch white corn tortillas, warmed (2 per serving)
- 1 cup mixed baby greens

INSTRUCTIONS

1 To make lentils, in a medium saucepan over medium heat, heat oil. Add onion and shallots; cook and stir 6 minutes or until tender. Stir in tomato paste, garlic powder, cumin and chili powder. Cook 1 minute. Add broth and lentils; bring to a boil. Reduce heat; gently simmer, uncovered, for 20 to 30 minutes, or until lentils are tender and cooked through. If necessary, drain excess liquid from lentils. Set aside.

2 Meanwhile, to roast cauliflower, preheat oven to 425°F. In a medium bowl, toss cauliflower florets with olive oil to lightly coat (you may not need all 3 tablespoons). Sprinkle with salt, black pepper and cayenne pepper. On a large rimmed baking sheets, arrange florets in a single layer. Roast 30 to 35 minutes or until golden on edges, tossing after 15 minutes.

3 For chipotle cream sauce, in a small bowl, combine mayonnaise, lime peel and juice, and adobo sauce or chipotle hot sauce. Season to taste with salt and pepper.

4 To assemble tacos, spoon lentil mixture on warm tortillas. Top with cauliflower and baby greens; drizzle with chipotle cream sauce.

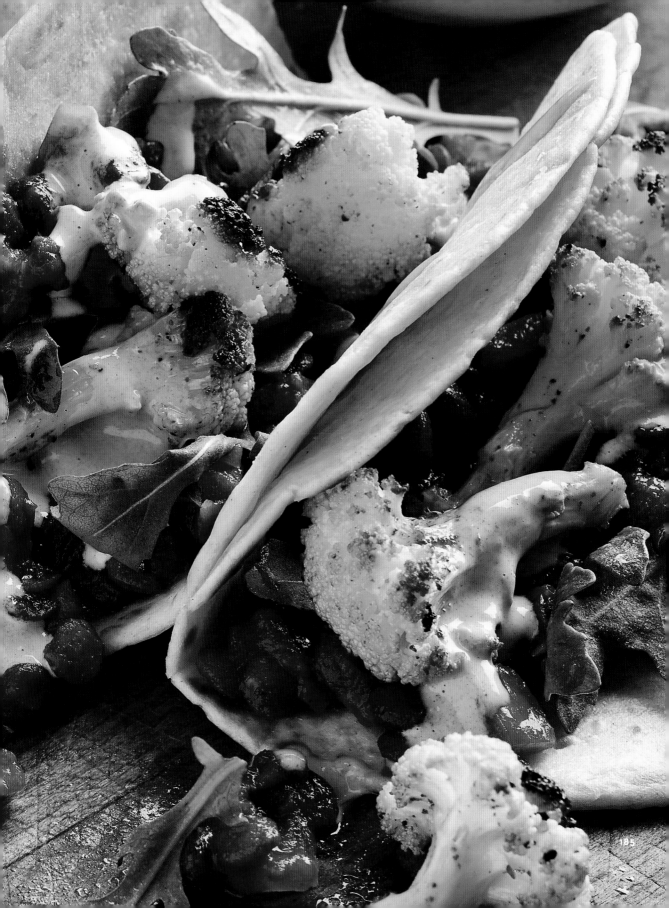

COVER Yelena Yemchuk/Getty Images **FRONT COVER FLAP** kate_sept2004/Getty Images **2–3** Yaroslav Danylchenko/500px **4–5** *From left:* Liam Franklin/Recipe styling and development: Margaret Monroe. All for you friend/Shutterstock. PeopleImages/Getty Images. Olena Rudo/500px/Getty Images **6–7** vaaseenaa/Getty Images **8–9** Melpomenem/Getty Images **10–11** vaaseenaa/Getty Images **12–13** istetiana/Getty Images **14–15** *From left:* Paul Bradbury/Getty Images. Lew Robertson/Getty Images **16–17** *From left:* Westend61/Getty Images. Lilechka75/Getty Images **18–19** *From left:* OatmealStories/Getty Images. fcafotodigital/Getty Images. © StockFood/Ivanova, Anna **20–21** PeopleImages/Getty Images **22–23** Megan Betteridge/Shutterstock **24–25** *From left:* PeopleImages/Getty Images. Orbon Alija/Getty Images **26–27** *From left:* Sarinya Pinngam/Getty Images. imaginima/Getty Images **28–29** Ivanko_Brnjakovic/Getty Images **30–31** *From left:* bigacis/Getty Images. PeopleImages/Getty Images **32–33** zarzamora/Shutterstock **34–35** Vera_Petrunina/Getty Images **36–37** All for you friend/Shutterstock **38–39** *From left:* Kolpakova Svetlana/Shutterstock. Davizro Photography/Shutterstock **40–41** *From left:* PicturePartners/Getty Images. Karissa/Getty Images **42–43** Lightspring/Shutterstock **44–45** ronstik/Getty Images **46–47** *From left:* Ponchai Soda/EyeEm/Getty Images. sveta_zarzamora/Getty Images **48–49** *From left:* See D Jan/Getty Images. nerudol/Getty Images **50–51** pixelfit/Getty Images **52–53** Sea Wave/Shutterstock **54–55** *From left:* RedHelga/Getty Images. VectorPot/Shutterstock **56–57** Si-Gal/Getty Images (2) **58–59** Si-Gal/Getty Images **60–61** Si-Gal/Getty Images **62–63** EasyBuy4u/Getty Images **64–65** Milaspage/Getty Images **66–67** Westend61/Getty Images **68–69** Westend61/Getty Images **70–71** filadendron/Getty Images **72–73** vgajic/Getty Images **74–75** Aleksandra Golubtsova/Getty Images **76–77** *Clockwise from top left:* sorendls/Getty Images. hh5800/Getty Images. hh5800/Getty Images. Suzifoo/Getty Images **78–79** Creativ Studio Heinemann/Getty Images **80–81** Creativ Studio Heinemann/Getty Images **82–83** iStock/Getty Images (2) **84–85** villagemoon/Getty Images **86–87** marekuliasz/Getty Images **88–89** *Clockwise from top left:* Altayb/Getty Images. PicturePartners/Getty Images. etienne voss/Getty Images. temmuzcan/Getty Images. baibaz/Getty Images. SashaHaltam/Getty Images **90–91** Natali Zakharova/Shutterstock **92–93** AS Food studio/Shutterstock **94–95** *From left:* Natali Zakharova/Shutterstock. Lauri Patterson/Getty Images **96–97** Pinkybird/Getty Images **98–99** Olena Rudo/500px/Getty Images **100–101** KristianSeptimius Krogh/Getty Images **102–103** kate_sept2004/Getty Images **104–105** Theerakul Ingkaninant/EyeEm/Getty Images **106–107** *From left:* Courtesy. Nina Firsova/Shutterstock **108–109** Natalia Klenova/EyeEm/Getty Images **110–111** Courtesy (2) **112–113** PeopleImages/Getty Images **114–115** PeopleImages/Getty Images **116–117** *Clockwise from top left:* zi3000/Getty Images. sveta_zarzamora/Getty Images. Alleko/Getty Images **118–119** Oleksandra Naumenko/Shutterstock **120–121** New Africa/Shutterstock **122–123** *From left:* gilaxia/Getty Images. Andrey Popov/Getty Images **124–125** Aleksandar Mijatovic/Shutterstock **126–127** 1989studio/Shutterstock **128–129** Anna Kolosyuk/Getty Images **130–131** Westend61/Getty Images **132–133** Tassii/Getty Images **134–135** knape/Getty Images **136–137** *From left:* The Good Brigade/Getty Images. PeopleImages/Getty Images **138–139** *Clockwise from left:* SolStock/Getty Images. manx_in_the_world/Getty Images. Monica Schipper/Getty Images. Frazer Harrison/Getty Images. C Flanigan/Getty Images. NBC/Getty Images. Valerie Macon/Getty Images **140–141** twomeows/Getty Images **142–143** Ken Carlson, Doug Samuelson/Food stylist: Joshua Hake **144–151** Liam Franklin/Recipe styling and development: Margaret Monroe (8) **152–153** Ken Carlson/Food stylist: Joshua Hake (2) **154–155** Liam Franklin/Recipe styling and development: Margaret Monroe **156–157** *From left:* Liam Franklin/Recipe styling and development: Margaret Monroe. Ken Carlson, Doug Samuelson/Food stylist: Joshua Hake **158–159** *From left:* Liam Franklin/Recipe styling and development: Margaret Monroe. Ken Carlson, Doug Samuelson/Food stylist: Joshua Hake **160–161** Ken Carlson, Doug Samuelson/Food stylist: Joshua Hake **162–163** Ken Carlson, Doug Samuelson/Food stylist: Joshua Hake **164–165** Ken Carlson/Food stylist: Joshua Hake **166–167** *From left:* Ken Carlson/Food stylist: Joshua Hake. Ken Carlson, Doug Samuelson/Food stylist: Joshua Hake **168–169** Liam Franklin/Recipe styling and development: Margaret Monroe **170–171** Alena Bugrova **172–173** Alena Bugrova **174–175** Ken Carlson, Doug Samuelson/Food stylist: Joshua Hake **176–177** Alena Bugrova **178–183** Liam Franklin/Recipe styling and development: Margaret Monroe (5) **184–185** Ken Carlson, Doug Samuelson/Food stylist: Joshua Hake **BACK COVER** *From top:* Lightfield Studios/Getty Images. Ken Carlson, Doug Samuelson/Food stylist: Joshua Hake. Melpomenem/Getty Images **BACK COVER FLAP** All for you friend/Shutterstock **SPINE** mariusFM77/Getty Images

SPECIAL THANKS TO CONTRIBUTING WRITERS

Dana Hudepohl

Janet Lee

Diana Kelly Levey

Margaret Monroe

Brittany Risher

Layla Shaffer

Michelle Stacey

Karla Walsh

DISCLAIMER Information in *Plant-Based for Tired People* is provided for awareness, education and general information. Health benefits of various diets, foods and weight-loss strategies are the opinion of the author, and there may be differing views on many of the topics covered, including evolving research, opinions, benefits and efficacy. This book is meant to inform the general reader and is not a substitute for medical advice by a physician, dietitian and/or nutritionist. Please consult a doctor if you have chronic ailments or feel adverse side effects after starting a nutrition regimen, and do not ingest items to which you have sensitivities or may be allergic. Readers should consult a licensed health professional who knows their personal medical history on matters relating to their health and well-being, including being aware of potential interactions with medications they are taking and conflicts with other wellness-related goals.

CENTENNIAL BOOKS

An Imprint of
Centennial Media, LLC
40 Worth St., 10th Floor
New York, NY 10013, U.S.A.

CENTENNIAL BOOKS is a trademark of Centennial Media, LLC

ISBN 978-1-951274-51-1

Distributed by
Simon & Schuster, Inc.
1230 Avenue of the Americas
New York, NY 10020, U.S.A.

For information about custom editions, special sales and premium and corporate purchases,
please contact Centennial Media at contact@centennialmedia.com.

Manufactured in China

10 9 8 7 6 5 4 3 2

Publishers & Co-Founders Ben Harris, Sebastian Raatz
Editorial Director Annabel Vered
Creative Director Jessica Power
Executive Editor Janet Giovanelli
Deputy Editors Ron Kelly, Alyssa Shaffer
Design Director Martin Elfers
Senior Art Director Pino Impastato
Art Directors Patrick Crowley, Natali Suasnavas, Joseph Ulatowski
Copy/Production Patty Carroll, Angela Taormina
Assistant Art Director Jaclyn Loney
Photo Editor April O'Neil
Production Manager Paul Rodina
Production Assistant Alyssa Swiderski
Editorial Assistant Tiana Schippa
Sales & Marketing Jeremy Nurnberg